Inherited Neurological Disorders

Zhi-Ying Wu

Editor

Inherited Neurological Disorders

Diagnosis and Case Study

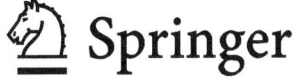 Springer

Editor
Zhi-Ying Wu
Department of Neurology and Research Center of Neurology
  Second Affiliated Hospital
Zhejiang University School of Medicine
Hangzhou
Zhejiang
China

ISBN 978-981-10-4195-2   ISBN 978-981-10-4196-9   (eBook)
DOI 10.1007/978-981-10-4196-9

Library of Congress Control Number: 2017946485

Printed on acid-free paper

This Springer imprint is published by Springer Nature
The registered company is Springer Nature Singapore Pte Ltd.
The registered company address is: 152 Beach Road, #21-01/04 Gateway East, Singapore 189721, Singapore

Contents

Yi Dong, Sheng Chen, Zhi-Jun Liu, Cong Lu, and Shi-Rui Gan

Abstract

Cerebellar ataxia can occur due to many diseases and manifest as diverse symptoms of failing to coordinate gait, balance, extremity, and eye movements. There are many causes of cerebellar ataxia; among others, genetic disorders are major causative factors. Hereditary ataxias are progressive, degenerative, and often fatal. Generally, the affected individuals ignore the disease status until they have children. In this chapter we introduced a subgroup of hereditary ataxias due to CAG repeat expansions in encoding and untranslated regions of the corresponding causative gene, including spinocerebellar ataxia (SCA) type 1, 2, 3, 6, 7, 12, and 17 and dentatorubral and pallidoluysian atrophy (DRPLA). Additionally, the relatively rare Gerstmann-Sträussler-Scheinker syndrome (GSS) and ataxia with oculomotor apraxia type 2 (AOA2) are presented here as well.

Keywords

SCA • DRPLA • GSS • AOA2 • Heterogeneity

Y. Dong (✉) • S. Chen • Z.-J. Liu • C. Lu
Department of Neurology and Research Center of Neurology, Second Affiliated Hospital, Zhejiang University School of Medicine, Hangzhou, China
e-mail: dongyi2242@hotmail.com

S.-R. Gan
Department of Neurology and Institute of Neurology, First Affiliated Hospital, Fujian Medical University, Fuzhou, China

© Springer Nature Singapore Pte Ltd. 2017
Z.-Y. Wu (ed.), *Inherited Neurological Disorders*, DOI 10.1007/978-981-10-4196-9_1

1.1 Spinocerebellar Ataxia Type 1 (SCA1)

A 36-Year-Old Male Presented with Gait Disturbance and Urine Incontinence

Clinical Presentations

A 36-year-old Chinese Han male was first presented in our Neurology Department with a 2-year history of slowly progressive gait disturbance and slurred speech and 1-year history of urine incontinence and sexual dysfunction. Based on his description, symptoms originated with awkwardness in both upper extremities, followed by gait disturbance. He felt the severe unsteadiness when going downstairs. Thereafter, he began to develop slurred speech with a plosive pitch. Currently, the main distresses severely affecting quality of life are urination urgency, hesitation, and erectile failure.

On examination, blood pressure was a little high, without orthostatic hypotension (supine blood pressure 125/100 mmHg, orthostatic blood pressure 120/100 mmHg at 3 min). Cranial nerve examination showed normal. The tendon reflexes of extremities were symmetrical increased (+++), but extensor plantar responses were negative. Dysarthria, with monotone and plosive articulation, was noted. However, dysphagia, nystagmus, and imbalance of saccade velocity were not observed, and his extraocular movements were normal. In addition, dysmetria were marked as well. Brain magnetic resonance imaging (MRI)

indicated the mild atrophy of cerebellum and brainstem (Fig. 1.1). His brother (III_5), aunt (II_4), uncle (II_5), and grandfather (I_1) underwent similar cerebellar deficits without autonomic nervous system abnormalities (Fig. 1.2).

Primary Diagnosis

The cerebellar deficits, dysautonomic presentations, and neurological examinations revealed the involvement of the cerebellum and autonomic nervous system. As for index patient, autonomic dys-

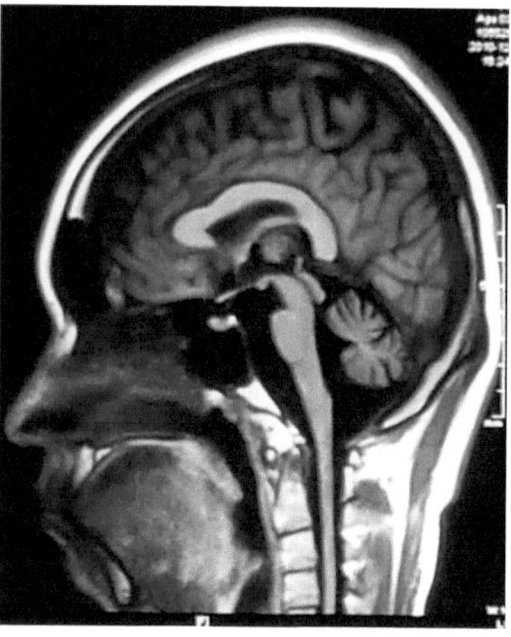

Fig. 1.1 Brain MRI of the index patient. A sagittal image demonstrates the mild atrophy of cerebellum and brainstem

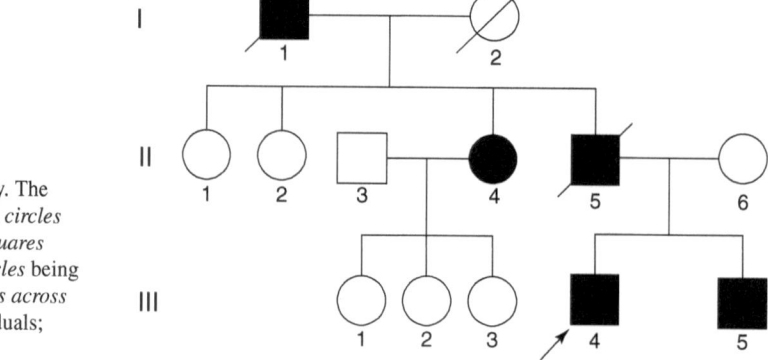

Fig. 1.2 Pedigree of the family. The *squares* indicate normal males; *circles* being normal females; *filled squares* being affected males; *filled circles* being affected females; *diagonal lines across symbols* being deceased individuals; *arrow* being the proband

function findings were followed by typical spinocerebellar ataxia presentations. We have excluded the secondary causes. The combination of dysautonomic expressions and cerebellar ataxia would be more typical of the cerebellar type of multiple system atrophy (MSA-C). Hence, MSA-C was impressed initially. However, positive family history, brain MRI, and neurological examination were suggestive of likely diagnosis of autosomal dominant cerebellar ataxia (ADCA). Based on Harding's classification, the proband could be categorized as ADCA type I, including spinocerebellar ataxia (SCA) types 1, 2, 3, 4, 12, 16, and 17 and DRPLA.

Additional Tests or Key Results

Autonomic failure in SCA patients has been reported successively recently [1–3]. Thus, according to the relative prevalence of SCA around the world [4], mutation analyses of *ATXN3* for SCA3, *ATXN2* for SCA2, and *ATXN1* for SCA1 were performed in the affected individuals, and the results showed to be negative in *ATXN3* and *ATXN2*, but positive in *ATXN1*. It has been identified that CAG repeat numbers of *ATXN1* are 28/47 in the proband (III$_4$) (Fig. 1.3) and 30/51 in his younger brother (III$_5$). The finding confirmed SCA1 diagnosis in this family.

Discussion

The onset of SCA1 is due to abnormal CAG repeat expansions within the causative gene, *ATXN1* [5]. The clinical picture of SCA1 patients is highly variable and mainly includes cerebellar ataxia, dysarthria, and eye movement abnormalities. Later in the disease, the further impairment of pontine could induce the occurrence of slow saccades and ophthalmoparesis. However, the phenotype barely helped to distinguish SCA1 from other SCA subtypes [6].

As regards the phenotype heterogeneity of SCA1, our current case manifested as unusual sexual dysfunction and urinary abnormality, which were uncharacteristic of SCA1 and not seen in the previous autonomic function investigation of SCA1 patients [2]. Compared to common occurrence of dysautonomic findings in SCA3 and SCA2 [1, 7], the autonomic complaints were seldom observed in patients with SCA1. The neuron degeneration in SCA1, despite most readily identified in the cerebellum and brainstem, involves widely in the whole brain and is responsible for the clinical profile. The previous neuropathology study has shown mild neuron loss of the cranial nerve nuclei including the vagi which regulates parasympathetic functions [8]. Thus, the dysautonomic findings of affected individual in our study could be connected with the involvement of autonomic nervous system.

So far, treatment of SCA1 patients is mainly supportive as no effective therapy to defer the disease progression. The previous studies have shown that intensive rehabilitation could improve motor coordination in a cohort of patients with cerebellar malfunction [9, 10]. Currently, intensive rehabilitation may be recommended for SCA1 patients since symptomatic improvement could cause the certain side effect.

Above all, this case expands the clinical profile of SCA1 and highlights that its clinical spectrum may be broader than previously considered. Moreover, SCA1 could be as a differential diagnosis of cases resembling MSA, especially those having dominant family history.

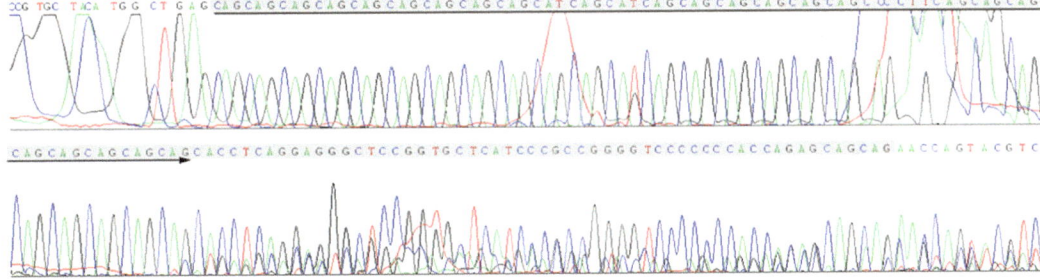

Fig. 1.3 Chromatogram of CAG repeats within *ATXN1* of the index patient (III$_4$). The *arrow* shows normal allele (28 CAG repeats), and the gray-highlighted sequence being expanded allele (47 CAG repeats)

1.2 Spinocerebellar Ataxia Type 2 (SCA2)

A 33-Year-Old Man Presented with Uncontrolled Movement of Head and Gait Disturbance

Clinical Presentations

A right-handed 33-year-old man presented to our Neurology Department with 6-year history of uncontrolled movement of head, 1-year history of slurred speech, 6-month history of gait disturbance, and occasionally swallowing difficulty when drinking. The affected individual first noted mild involuntary movement affecting his head at 27 years of age. Over the next 4–5 years, this distress worsened progressively. Four years later speech disorder developed, followed by unsteady gait, causing to fall down especially when running, and swallowing difficulty when drinking. He was not yet treated when consulting us. There was no disease history of brain trauma, encephalitis, and exposure history to dopamine-blocking agents or alcohol. His father (II$_1$) and grandmother (I$_2$) underwent resembling symptoms without uncontrolled movement of head.

Neurologic examinations revealed dysarthria, limb, and gait ataxia. Cranial nerve examinations showed slow saccadic eye movement and ophthalmoplegia of abduction. His muscle force, tension, and sensory reactions were normal. The decreased or absent tendon reflexes were observed. The ataxia signs comprising finger-nose test, rapid alternating movements, and heel-knee-shin test all indicated the cerebellar malfunction. Brain magnetic resonance imaging (MRI) of the index patient demonstrated the mild atrophy of cerebellum (Fig. 1.4).

Primary Diagnosis

This was an adolescent man with cerebellar ataxia manifestations and involuntary movement of head. The phenotype revealed the impairment of cerebellum and extrapyramidal tract.

Currently, the index case mainly experienced involuntary movement of head, accompanied by cerebellar ataxia signs. According to the previous study [11], Huntington's disease (HD) was

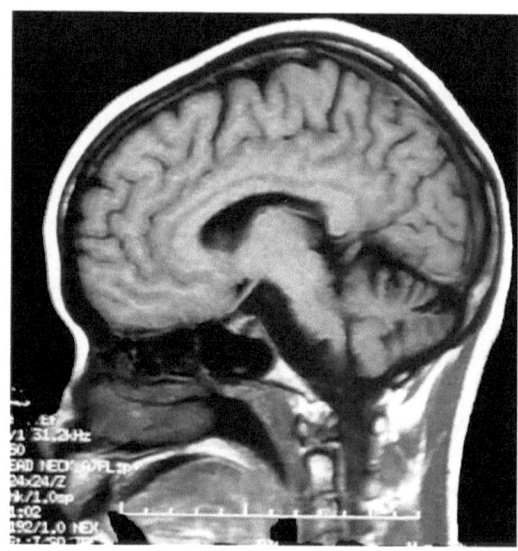

Fig. 1.4 Brain MRI of the index patient. A sagittal image demonstrates the mild atrophy of cerebellum

possible, but the typical presentations including psychiatric and behavior disorders and cognitive impairment were absent. In order to exclude the probability, we carried out *HTT* gene screening for the affected individuals. However, this causative gene of HD was negative for the affected family members.

Additional Tests or Key Results

Hereditary anticipation was noted in this family, and onset age of the proband's father began in the sixth decade with slow disease progression (Fig. 1.5). Combined with the common ataxia symptoms among family members, brain MRI, and neurological examination, autosomal dominant cerebellar ataxia (ADCA) should be highly suspected. Based on Harding's classification, the index patient could be diagnosed as ADCA type I, including spinocerebellar ataxia (SCA) types 1, 2, 3, 4, 12, 16, and 17 and DRPLA.

Furthermore, slow saccadic eye movement and ophthalmoplegia of abduction, as clinical hallmarks of SCA2 compared to other SCA subtypes, were observed as well in the index patient. In order to confirm diagnosis, we screened *ATXN2* mutation for the proband (III$_1$) and demonstrated that he carried 22/45 CAG repeats within *ATXN2* (Fig. 1.6), which confirmed the diagnosis of SCA2.

Discussion

SCA2 is induced by an abnormal CAG expansion within *ATXN2* and mainly characterized by slowly progressive ataxia gait, dysphagia, dysarthria, ophthalmoplegia, and polyneuropathy [12, 13]. It is the next most common SCA subtype around the world, only exceeded by SCA3 [4]. Despite SCA2 shares clinical expressions with other SCA subtypes, a slow saccadic eye movement represents its clinical marker, which is distinct from other common SCA phenotypes [14].

SCAs could manifest as a large variety of non-cerebellar symptoms, including various combinations of hyperkinetic and hypokinetic movement defects. During the disease course of various SCA subtypes, movement disorder could be the presenting, prominent, or even solitary disease characteristics [15]. SCA2 is prone to express typical extrapyramidal signs, including parkinsonism, dystonia, and myoclonus. Only a few cases have been reported to present with choreiform movements in SCA2 [16–18]. Our case firstly reported that SCA2 could present with HD phenocopy in China.

The related clinical tests of SCA2 are very finite due to the rare SCA2 patients and complicated clinical manifestations [19]. However, the clinical improvements in certain disease presentations have been described. For instance, the effective subthalamic-thalamic deep brain stimulation (DBS) could alleviate postural tremor of SCA2 patients [20], whereas dopaminergic and anticholinergics drugs have also been observed to improve movement disorder in SCA2 patients [21]. Altogether, despite neither medicine nor physical therapy could delay the disease progression notably, the helpful treatment has been shown to improve quality of life.

In conclusion, we described a SCA2 patient overlapping with clinical manifestations of HD. In the future, when confronted with an affected individual with involuntary movement, that is, combined with cerebellar ataxia, we should screen for SCA2 mutation under the condition of negative results of well-known causative genes.

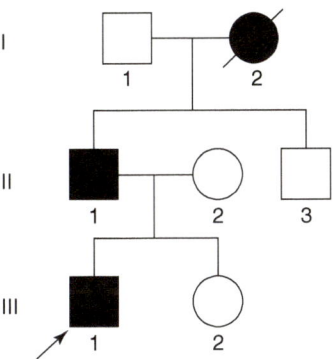

Fig. 1.5 Pedigree chart of the family. The *squares* demonstrate males; *circles* being females; *filled squares* being affected males; *filled circle* being affected female; *diagonal line* across symbol being the deceased individual; *arrow* being the index patient

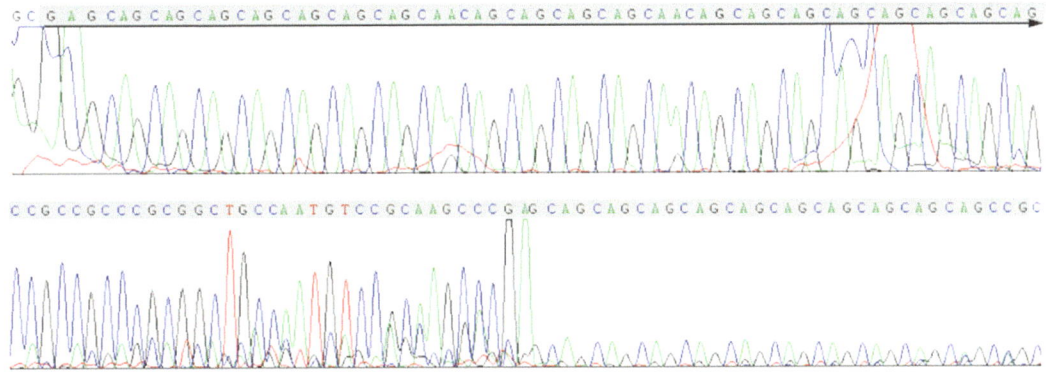

Fig. 1.6 Chromatogram of CAG repeats within *ATXN2* in the index patient (III₁). The *arrow* indicates normal allele (22 CAG repeats); the *gray-highlighted sequence* indicates the expanded allele (45 CAG repeats)

1.3 Spinocerebellar Ataxia Type 3 (SCA3)

A 57-Year-Old Woman Presented with Ataxia and Peripheral Neuropathy

Clinical Presentations

A 57-year-old Chinese woman came to the clinic with an 8-year history of unstable gait, 2-year history of slurred speech, and swallowing difficulty. She had no remarkable past medical history. Her father (I_1), brother (II_5), daughter (III_1), and niece (IV_4) had the resembling manifestations as well (Fig. 1.7).

On examination, she had no abnormal cranial nerves signs other than saccadic eye movement on pursuit. The muscular force and tension were intact. There was no sensory deficit except for the right lower extremities. Its sensory abnormalities included hypopselaphesia, diminished vibration, and position sense. The tendon reflexes of upper limbs were absent, while lower limbs were normal. Babinski sign was negative. Eye movement recording showed horizontal nystagmus. Ataxia signs of limbs and trunk were noted, including positive finger-nose and heel-knee-shin tests.

Her electromyography (EMG) investigation disclosed the mild reduction of amplitude of compound sensory action potential, indicating axonal neuropathy in her four limbs. The brain magnetic resonance image (MRI) showed the cerebellar atrophy (Fig. 1.8).

Primary Diagnosis

The clinical presentations, neurological examinations, brain MRI, and EMG data showed that the comprehensive involvement of cerebellum and peripheral nerve.

During the whole disease course, cerebellar ataxia was the prominent presentation. Combined with noted family history, autosomal dominant cerebellar ataxia (ADCA) was firstly considered. Specifically, due to the elder age of onset and slow disease progression, spinocerebellar ataxia (SCA) type 6 should be strongly suspected among the affected family members. However, genetic screening for *CACNA1A*, which is the causative gene of SCA6, was negative and excluded the initial diagnosis.

Additional Tests or Key Results

Besides typical cerebellar ataxia presentations, peripheral neuropathy should be noted during

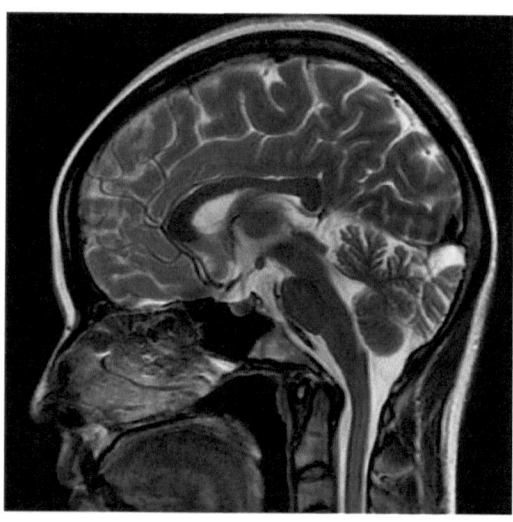

Fig. 1.8 Brain magnetic resonance imaging in the index patient. A T2-weighted sagittal image demonstrates the cerebellum atrophy

Fig. 1.7 Pedigree chart of the family. *The squares* demonstrate males; *circles* being females; *filled squares* being affected males; *filled circles* being affected females; *diagonal line* across symbol being the deceased individual; *arrow* being the index patient

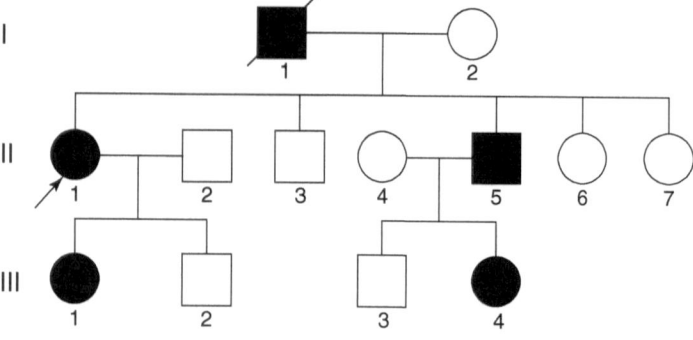

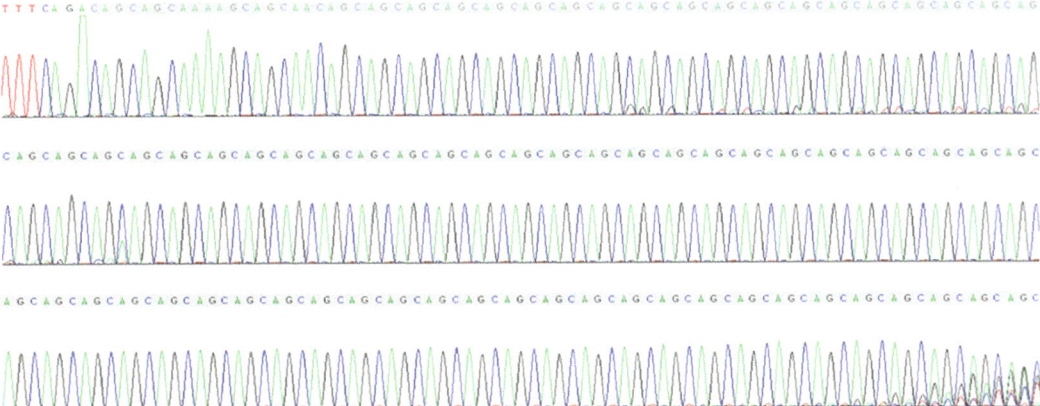

Fig. 1.9 Chromatogram of CAG repeats within *ATXN3* in the index patient. The *gray-highlighted sequence* indicates the expanded allele with 79 CAG repeats

disease course. Peripheral neuropathy has long been recognized in SCA3 patients. Moreover, due to the highest prevalence of SCA3 in China, we further screened for this subtype. After carrying out genetic study of CAG repeat within *ATXN3* gene of the index patient, it was identified that the CAG repeat copies within abnormal allele were 79 (Fig. 1.9), confirming SCA3 diagnosis in this family.

Discussion

SCA3, also termed as Machado-Joseph disease (MJD), is the most prevalent subtype of SCA across the globe [4] and the highest prevalence in China as well [22]. It is induced by CAG copy expansions within exon 10 of *ATXN3* gene on chromosome 14q32.1 [23]. The disease onset is typically in the second and fourth decade, and its clinical profile mainly includes cerebellar ataxia and a various combination of pyramidal and extrapyramidal signs, cognitive impairment, and neuropathies [24].

SCA3 has the noted clinical phenotype diversity and generally shares clinical manifestations with other SCA subtypes. Based upon this phenotypic variability, Portuguese researchers classified SCA3 into four types [25]. Type 1 disease has features of prominent dystonic-rigid syndrome and early onset, often with little ataxia; type 2, marked unsteady posture and gait and intermediate onset; type 3, cerebellar dysfunction,

peripheral neuropathy, and late onset; and type 4, obvious presentations of Parkinson's disease and variable onset. Besides, SCA3 patients also presented as spastic paraplegia without ataxia signs [26–28], it is advised to be the fifth type. The five clinical subtypes could transform reciprocally during disease course, or two or more clinical subtypes coexist in one patient simultaneously [29].

In view of presenting symptoms of the index patient, including late onset and peripheral neuropathy, she could be impressed in type 3. The previous studies demonstrated a different degree of involvement of peripheral nerve in SCA3 patients, especially frequent among patients with late onset [30]. Distal axonal neuropathy has also been observed in a large cohort of SCA3 patients, either histopathologically or electrophysiologically [31–33]. Further study suggested that neuropathy basis is due to loss of myelinated and unmyelinated fibers [34].

So far, there is no medication to slow disease course of SCA3. Therefore, the systematic preventions of secondary complications seem to be preferable to patients, including vitamin supplements, regular physical activity, weight control, etc. Altogether, SCA3 should be suspected in patient presenting with late-onset ataxia and polyneuropathy of unknown etiology. It should be considered as a rare differential diagnosis of polyneuropathy with family history.

1.4 Spinocerebellar Ataxia Type 6 (SCA6)

A 49-Year-Old Female Presented with Gait Disturbance and Dysarthria

Clinical Presentations

A 49-year-old woman complained about 2 years of gait disturbance accompanied by episodic vertigo and dysarthria in our clinic. She also felt nausea and vomited occasionally during vertigo attack. She didn't report any manifestations of diplopia and muscle weakness. Her neurological examination revealed mild horizontal gaze-evoked nystagmus and slurred speech. Cranial nerve examinations revealed normal visual acuity, visual fields, and extraocular movements. The examination of muscles was also unremarkable. Her bilateral knee reflexes were symmetrically increased (+++) and Babinski signs were negative. She also showed positive heel-knee-tibia test and Romberg's sign. Brain MRI revealed severe cerebellar atrophy (Fig. 1.10). The patient's mother suffered with similar symptoms in her late 40s and died at age 75 (Fig. 1.11). Other medical history of the patient was unremarkable.

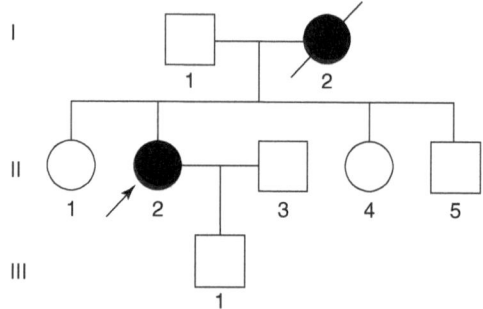

Fig. 1.11 Pedigree chart of the family. *The squares* show males; *circles* being females; *filled circles* being affected females; *diagonal line across symbol* being the deceased individual; *arrow* being the index patient

Primary Diagnosis

Based on the pure cerebellar symptoms, neurological examinations and brain MRI, the localization most likely involves the cerebellum. The involvement of the cerebral cortex and spinal cord was much less likely. The late-onset symptoms and autosomal dominant inheritance pattern remind a diagnosis of autosomal dominant cerebellar ataxia (ADCA). Based upon the Harding's classification, this patient should be diagnosed with ADCA type III. It comprises several subtypes of spinocerebellar ataxias (SCAs), including SCA5, SCA6, SCA11, SCA26, SCA30, and SCA31. Among them, SCA6 is the most common subtype [35]. Therefore, a *CACNA1A* gene test for SCA6 was then arranged.

Additional Tests or Key Results

Gene test revealed a prolonged expansion of trinucleotide repeats (25 CAG repeats) in *CACNA1A* gene (Fig. 1.12).

Discussion

SCA6 is a late-onset neurodegenerative disorder characterized by relatively pure cerebellar ataxia accompanied by eye movement disturbances, such as gaze-evoked nystagmus, abnormal smooth pursuit, and vestibulo-ocular reflex [36]. It was induced by CAG repeat expansion within exon 49 of the *CACNA1A* gene.

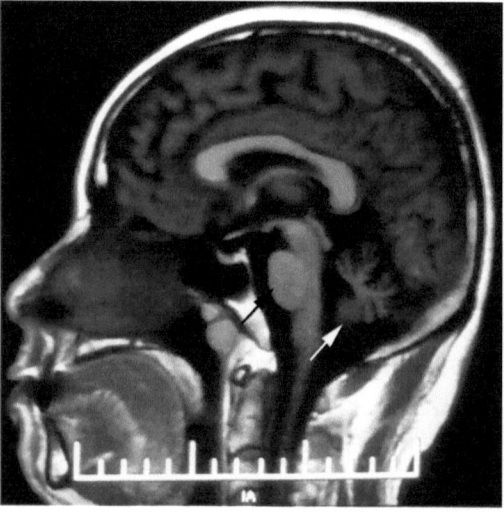

Fig. 1.10 T1-weighted sagittal MRI image of the patient. The *white arrow* points to severe cerebellar atrophy. The *black arrow* points to relatively spared pons

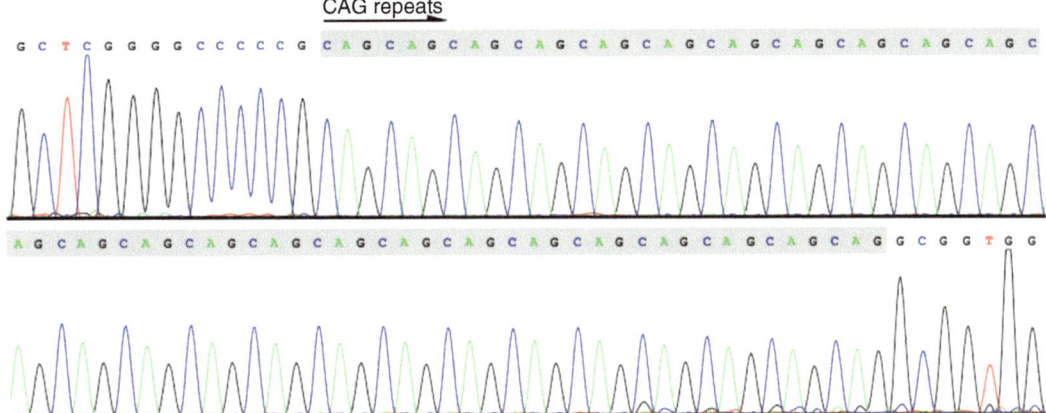

Fig. 1.12 Sequencing chromatogram of the expanded CAG copies (25 repeats) of the affected individual

The natural history of SCA6 can be very long. Several reports suggested that patient can even walk without stumbling up to 20 years after disease onset [37–39]. It has also been demonstrated that about 60% of patients develop illness after 50 years old. Anticipation was frequently reported in SCAs. However, it has not been observed in SCA6, which might be due to a relatively small pathogenic expansion range (usually 19–29) [36, 40–42].

The involvement scope of brain damage in SCA6 is basically similar to which in other types of SCAs. However, it mainly restricts in the brain regions of the motor cerebellothalamocortical loop, whereas the motor basal ganglia-thalamo-cortical loop seems to be relatively intact [43]. It has been previously revealed that subcortical neurotransmitter systems remain spared during neurodegenerative process of SCA6 except for the midbrain dopaminergic substantia nigra [44].

To date, there is no cure for SCAs, including SCA6. However, several clinical trials have been conducted. One study suggested that acetazolamide (250–500 mg/day) can temporally but significantly improve the postural sway in SCA6 patients [45]. Unfortunately, the improvement became weaker after 1 year [45]. Other drugs like buspirone and tandospirone have been proven effective to improve the mean global ataxia score or International Cooperative Ataxia Rating Scale (ICARS) in several clinical trials [46–48]. Besides, latest results of a randomized, double-blind, placebo-controlled trial supported that riluzole could be a promising treatment for cerebellar ataxia, whereas its application in SCA6 and underlying mechanism remain unknown [49].

1.5 Spinocerebellar Ataxia Type 7 (SCA7)

A 22-Year-Old Girl Presented with Ataxia and Visual Dysfunction

Clinical Presentations

The patient is a 22-year-old Han Chinese girl. At approximately 17 years of age, she first felt gait imbalance and lower extremity weakness, especially when walking. Thereafter, the slurred speech and visual dysfunction were progressively noted. Sometimes, she also suffered from swallowing difficulty when eating and drinking. At that time, she was diagnosed as ataxia disorder. However, she did not accept any treatment until now. She had no remarkable past medical history. The successive pregnancy, birth, and postpartum were ordinary.

On admission, she was conscious and dysarthric. Eye examinations showed the relatively normal visual acuity and field. The color discrimination displayed the mild impairment. The cranial nerve examinations showed no other abnormalities. Muscle strength and tendon reflexes were intact, and bilateral Babinski signs were negative. The mild muscular hypertonia was observed in her lower extremities. Sensory system was normal. Finger-nose and heel-knee-shin tests were remarkably abnormal.

Magnetic resonance imaging (MRI) of the brain showed normal (Fig. 1.13a). However, the mild atrophy of thoracic spinal cord was observed (Fig. 1.13b). There were 7 affected family members in three consecutive generations. Her mother (II_4) and younger sister (III2) had similar symptoms, with the first onset age of 32 and 7 years, respectively (Fig. 1.14).

Primary Diagnosis

The cerebellar ataxia presentations and thoracic spinal cord atrophy indicated the involvement of cerebellum and spinal cord. Combined with autosomal dominant inheritance mode and noted

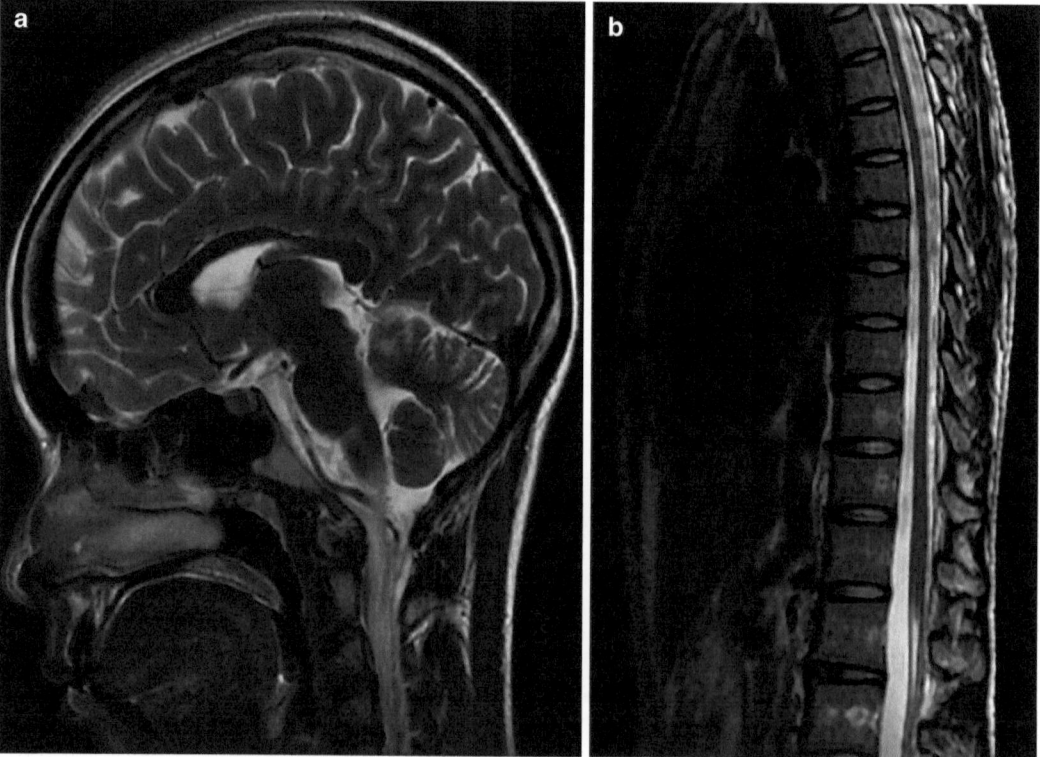

Fig. 1.13 Magnetic resonance imaging scan of brain and spinal cord of the proband. (**a**) T2-weighted sagittal image demonstrates the normal brain. (**b**) The mild atrophy of thoracic spinal cord was observed

Fig. 1.14 Pedigree of the family. *The squares* represent males; *circles* being females; *filled squares* being affected males; *filled circles* being affected females; *diagonal lines across symbols* being deceased individuals; *arrow* being the proband

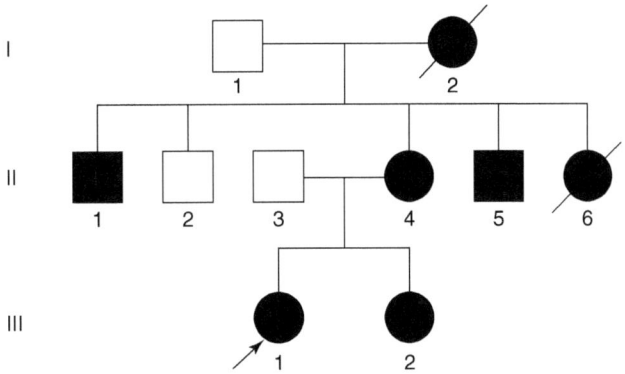

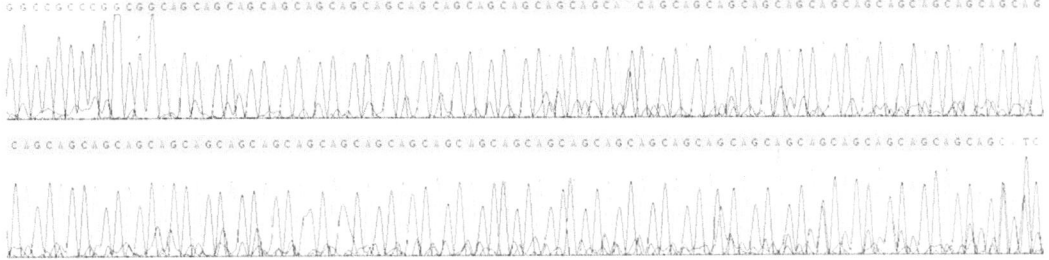

Fig. 1.15 Chromatogram of CAG repeats within *ATXN7* of the index patient. The *gray-highlighted sequence* indicates the expanded allele with 56 CAG repeats

genetic anticipation, the diagnosis of spinocerebellar ataxia (SCA) could be made. Moreover, the proband and affected family members had progressive visual dysfunction. Therefore, the diagnosis of SCA7 should be firstly considered.

As for differential diagnosis, other common subtypes of SCA and mitochondrial encephalopathies such as NARP (neurogenic muscle weakness, ataxia, and retinitis pigmentosa) should be suspected as well. A few cases with SCA1, SCA2, and SCA3 have been observed to manifest as progressive visual loss [50–52]. And some individuals with NARP can present with ataxia and optic nerve degeneration [53]. Therefore, gene analysis of *ATXN7*, as causative gene of SCA7, needs to be carried out to confirm the diagnosis.

Additional Tests or Key Results

The CAG repeat copies existing in exon 3 of *ATXN7* were amplified via PCR, and the PCR product was electrophoresed and sequenced. It was identified that the CAG repeat copies within abnormal allele were 56 (Fig. 1.15), confirming SCA7 diagnosis in this family.

Discussion

SCA7 is a relatively common SCA subtype. It is also known as autosomal dominant cerebellar ataxia type II (ADCA-II), based upon Harding's classification [54]. The prevalence of SCA7 varies among different ethnic groups. It is the most prevalent subtype in South Africa, Mexico, and the Scandinavian countries such as Sweden and Finland. SCA7 is induced by a CAG repeat expansion existing in exon 3 of the *ATXN7* gene on chromosome 3p14-21.1 [55]. The CAG repeat copy number is 4–35 in normal individuals while 38–406 in SCA7 patients and inversely correlated with onset age. It will cause very rare infantile-onset cases (onset age less than 2 years) when CAG repeat number is beyond 130 [56]. The clinical manifestations of SCA7 include progressive cerebellar ataxia, dysarthria, dysphagia, decreased visual acuity, and color blindness in the blue-yellow axis. For the treatment, there are no effective drugs for SCA7 patients so far.

SCA7 has similar clinical manifestations with other common SCA subtypes. However, it also has some distinguished clinical features such as visual symptoms and pronounced genetic anticipation. Visual symptoms, including color blindness in the blue-yellow axis, abnormality in central visual acuity, hemeralopia, and photophobia, are caused by optic nerve atrophy and pigmental macular dystrophy. Almost all the SCA7 cases develop visual abnormalities during disease course. It is important to know that visual symptoms may precede, accompany, or follow the onset of ataxia [57]. Just like the index patient, visual symptoms could be accompanied by normal or subtle ophthalmoscopic findings and ataxia.

The marked anticipation due to further expansion of CAG repeats on transmission in successive generations is another hallmark of SCA7. The anticipation was more obvious during paternal transmission and could lead to some infantile-onset cases. There were some characteristic manifestations of infantile SCA7 cases comparing to the adult-onset patients [58, 59]. Firstly, infantile cases generally carried larger than 130 CAG repeats. Secondly, most of them had clinical expressions consisting of hypotonia and multiorgan damage such as patent ductus arteriosus, respiratory distress, capillary leak syndrome, renal dysfunction, and hepatomegaly. Thirdly, the overall survival was very short and less than 8 months in most cases. In summary, this is a typical SCA7 pedigree and shares the common disease presentations with other reported SCA7 cases.

1.6   Spinocerebellar Ataxia Type 12 (SCA12)

A 61-Year-Old Woman Presented with Action Tremor and Ataxia

Clinical Presentations

The proband (II$_6$) is a 61-year-old, right-handed woman who was otherwise healthy when, at age 51, she developed the involuntary head movement, especially being nervous or fatigue. The frequency and amplitude of head tremor aggravated progressively. During the next 7 years, she developed postural and kinetic tremor in her limbs. Currently, her upright posture became unstable and manifested as a broad-based and staggering gait. She sought medical care in a local hospital and was diagnosed with essential tremor. Thereafter, the unknown Chinese medicine cure was started, and symptoms could be approved moderately according to her statement. The affected family members, including her father (I$_1$) and brother (II$_2$), also presented with uncontrolled movement and gait disturbance (Fig. 1.16).

Symptoms slowly aggravated and she was examined at age 61. There was no oculomotor abnormality and nystagmus. The action tremor of head and limbs were observed. Dysarthria is noted during her overall disease course. There was no pyramidal weakness or sensory abnormality. Muscle tone was increased in all four limbs. The ataxia examinations including finger-nose test, rapid alternating movements, and heel-to-shin test all showed defective

condition of the cerebellum. Magnetic resonance imaging test, which was performed at age 61, displayed cerebellum atrophy (Fig. 1.17).

Primary Diagnosis

Gait imbalance and ataxia presentations revealed the involvement of cerebellum. Cerebellar signs were obvious in the index patient, further indicating that the impairment of central nervous system mainly refers to the cerebellum.

The characteristic clinical symptoms and signs comprise poorly coordinated gait, dysarthria, and positive family history of ataxia. Therefore, the

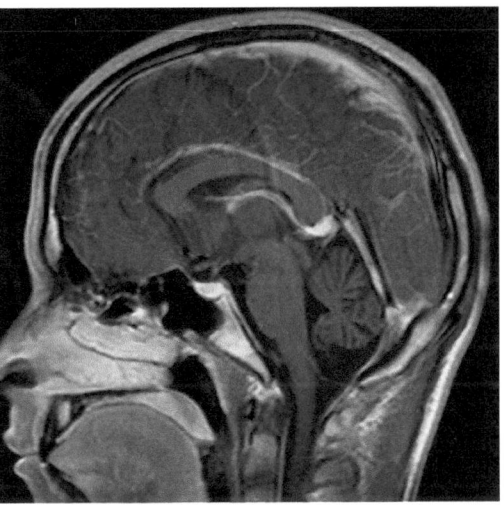

Fig. 1.17 Magnetic resonance imaging scan of brain in the index patient. A sagittal image demonstrates cerebellum atrophy

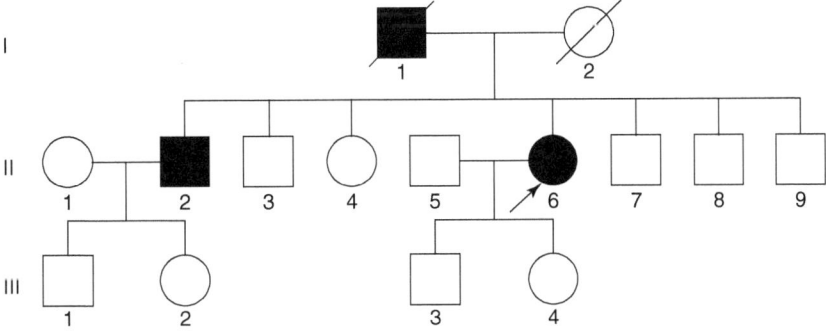

Fig. 1.16 Pedigree chart of the family. The *squares* represent males; *circles* being females; *filled squares* or *circles* being affected individuals; *diagonal lines across symbols* being the deceased individuals; *arrows* being the index patient

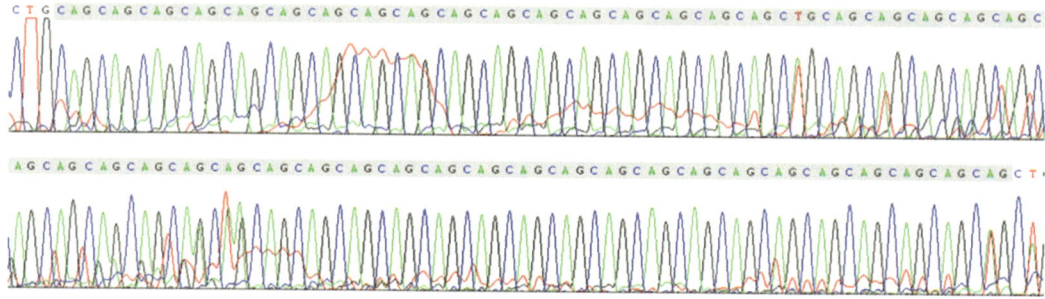

Fig. 1.18 Chromatogram of CAG repeats within *PPP2R2B* in the index patient. The *gray-highlighted sequence* indicates the expanded allele with 47 CAG repeats

affected patients could be established as the diagnosis of autosomal dominant cerebellar ataxia (ADCA) type I, including spinocerebellar ataxia (SCA) types 1, 2, 3, 4, 12, 16, and 17 and DRPLA.

Additional Tests or Key Results

According to the prevalence of SCA in China, we firstly screened for the four common SCA subtypes, including SCA3, SCA2, SCA1, and SCA6 [60]. The genetic screening results showed to be negative. In addition, action tremor could serve as clinical hallmark of SCA12 compared to other SCA subtypes. Therefore, as the causative gene of SCA12, *PPP2R2B* gene test was further performed for the index patient. Genetic result was abnormal with CAG repeat expansion in one allele, consistent with a diagnosis of SCA12. Specifically, II_6 harbored 47 CAG copies within disease allele (Fig. 1.18).

Discussion

SCA12 is characterized by onset of action tremor of body part, slowly followed by cerebellar ataxia and cortical signs [61]. *PPP2R2B* is the only causative gene of SCA12, and abnormal expansions of CAG repeats within *PPP2R2B* ultimately induce disease onset [62].

In the current case, we confirmed CAG repeat expansion within *PPP2R2B* gene of the proband and available family members. The prevalence of SCA12 is quite low across the world. Only a few SCA12 pedigrees have been reported in the literature. Besides several Indian cases due to likely founder effect [61, 63, 64], other SCA12 cases were detected in the USA, Singapore, Italy, and China [62, 65–68].

The noted clinical presentation distinct from other SCA subtypes is action tremor of the head and/or hands, preceding ataxia presentations. Although tremors as part of cerebellar syndrome are common in SCA, this type of tremor is only the condition of cerebellar malfunction and is closed to ataxia severity. Contrarily, the proband initially developed action tremor of the head. With the progress of the disease, tremor involved her limbs.

In contrast to SCA3, SCA1, and SCA2, SCA12 has the relatively slow progression and may not have a negative impact on longevity. Currently, there are few systemic studies on therapy, and only symptomatic treatment is available for tremor. The use of beta-blockers, clonazepam, and primidone has been proved to decrease tremor amplitude to improve life quality [69].

In summary, an affected individual with action tremor, slow disease progression, and dominant ataxia family history is strongly indicative of SCA12 and should be given to *PPP2R2B* genetic screening.

1.7 Spinocerebellar Ataxia Type 17 (SCA17)

A 45-Year-Old Female Presented with Gait Disturbance and Mood Changes

Clinical Presentations

A 45-year-old woman presented to our clinic complaining of 4 years of gait disturbance and difficulties in grasping stuff with her both hands. She developed slurred speech as well as swallowing problems 2 years ago. She also claimed to have a 1-year history of memory loss and mood changes. Besides, the patient denied seizures and hearing problems during her disease course. And, there was no history of fever, autoimmune diseases, blood clots, or miscarriages.

On neurological examinations, her vital signs were notable for speech and swallowing difficulties, increased muscle tone, tendon hyperreflexia with positive bilateral Hoffmann signs and Babinski signs, as well as several beats of bilateral ankle clonus. Her gait was slightly wide based and she had difficulties in walking straight. Additionally, her finger-nose test and heel-knee-tibia tests were positive, while Romberg sign was negative. All cranial nerve examinations revealed normal. The examination of muscle strength and sensory system including pinprick, light touch, temperature, vibration, and proprioception was also unremarkable. She scored 18 in the Scale for the Assessment and Rating of Ataxia (SARA) and 25 in Mini-Mental State Examination (MMSE). Brain MRI showed the obvious atrophy of her cerebellum, pons, and medulla (Fig. 1.19). Her family history revealed that several family members presented with similar symptoms as well (Fig. 1.20).

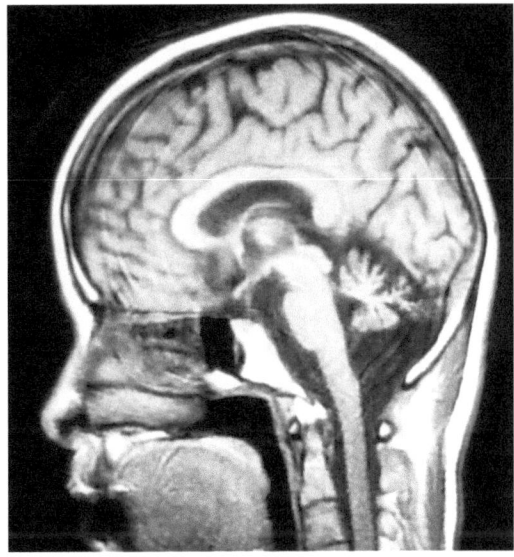

Fig. 1.19 T1-weighted sagittal brain MRI revealed the obvious atrophy of cerebellum, pons, and medulla

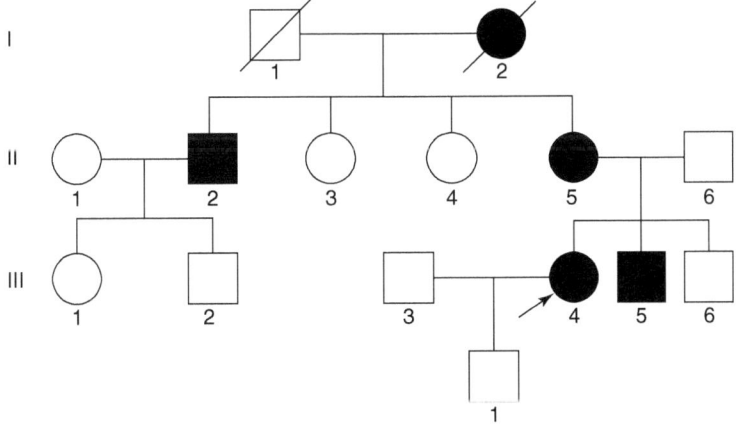

Fig. 1.20 Pedigree chart of the family. The *squares* represent males; circles being females; filled squares or circles being affected individuals; diagonal lines across symbols being the deceased individuals; arrows being the index patient

Primary Diagnosis

The patient's difficulties in walking and grasping stuff as well as positive finger-nose test and heel-knee-tibia test remind that the localization most likely involves the cerebellum, brainstem, as well as spinal cord. The negative findings in sensory system examination ruled out the possibility of sensory ataxia. The complaints of memory loss and mood changes together with mild abnormality in MMSE remind that the localization might also involve the cerebral cortex. Her increased muscle tone and tendon hyperreflexia, positive Hoffmann signs, and Babinski signs as well as bilateral ankle clonus revealed an involvement of bilateral pyramidal tracts. Her brain MRI suggested an atrophy of cerebellum, pons, and medulla, which was consistent with her symptomatologic and neurological examinations' localization. The patient's family history and inheritance pattern hinted a diagnosis of autosomal dominant cerebellar ataxia (ADCA). According to Harding's classification, she was diagnosed with ADCA type I, which comprises a series of spinocerebellar ataxias (SCAs) plus other neurological signs. The most common ADCA type I is SCA3 followed by SCA2 and SCA1, in descending order. Given a fact that SCA3 merely involves the cerebral cortex, SCA12 usually presents with obvious action tremor and dentatorubral-pallido-luysian atrophy (DRPLA) with progressive myoclonic epilepsy. Therefore, gene tests for SCA1, SCA2, and SCA17 were arranged.

Additional Tests or Key Results

Gene tests for SCA1 and SCA2 were all negative. Gel electrophoresis of exon 3 of *TBP* gene suggested a pathogenic expanded allele (Fig. 1.21a). Sequencing of the PCR fragment revealed a 49 CAG trinucleotide repeat expansion (Fig. 1.21b).

Discussion

SCA17 is a dominant inherited neurodegenerative disorder characterized by cerebellar ataxia, neuropsychiatric symptoms, and involuntary movements, including chorea and dystonia. It is caused by an expanded CAG trinucleotide repeats in exon 3 of TATA box-binding protein gene (*TBP*) [70, 71]. The TATA-Box-binding protein (TBP) is the most important component of the initiation complex of eukaryotic RNA polymerases [72]. A previous study suggested that there were several CAA interruptions within the CAG repeats, while CAG repeats with no CAA interruption showed increased instability [73].

It has been reported that about 1% of likely Huntington's disease (HD) cases are actually HD-like (HDL) [74]. HDL includes HDL1, HDL2, HDL3, and HDL4, DRPLA, neuroferritinopathy, benign hereditary chorea, and Wilson's disease (Table 1.1). SCA17, also termed as HDL4, can mimic phenotypes of HD, especially involuntary movements [75]. An integrated data including 122 patients from 55 pedigrees have demonstrated that dementia is the second most

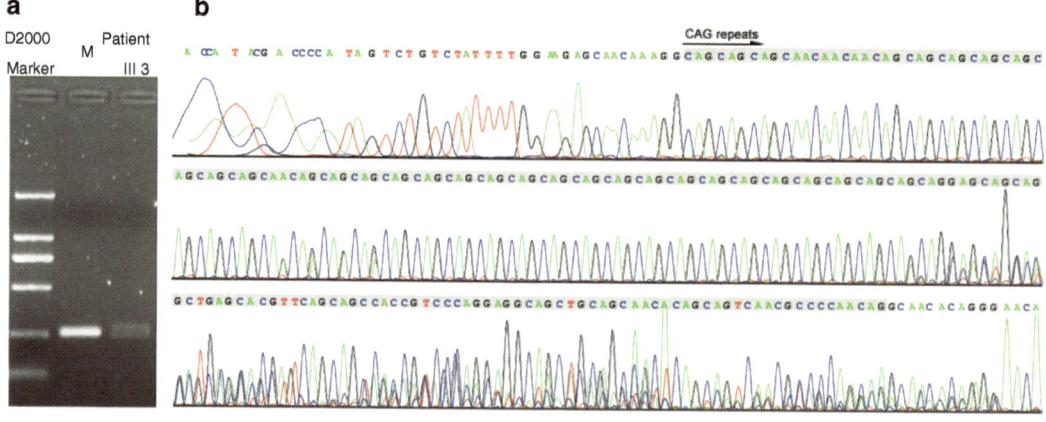

Fig. 1.21 Mutation analysis of the patient. (**a**) The agarose gel electrophoresis of the PCR fragment containing expanded CAG repeats. (**b**) Sequencing chromatogram of the expanded CAG repeats of the patient

Table 1.1 Summary of important autosomal dominant disorder cause of chorea syndromes

Condition	Inheritance	Gene	Mutation types	Age at onset	Clinical features
HD	AD	*HTT*	CAG repeats	<30	Chorea, dementia, psychiatric symptom
HDL1	AD	*PRNP*	Point mutation	20–45	Similar to HD with prominent personality change
HDL2	AD	*JPH3*	CAG/CTG repeats	25–45	Similar to HD, most frequent in black South Africans of sub-Saharan descent
HDL3	AR	–		3–4	Resembling juvenile HD, only described in two Saudi-Arabian families
HDL4 (SCA17)	AD	*TBP*	CAG repeats	3–75	Ataxia and HD phenocopy
DRPLA	AD	*ATN1*	CAG repeats	20–30	Severe progressive myoclonus epilepsy and cognitive decline in juveniles, while ataxia, choreoathetosis, and dementia in adults
Neuroferritinopathy	AD	*FTL1*	Point mutation	40s	Chorea, dystonia, oromandibular, etc.
Benign hereditary chorea	AD	*TITF-1*	Point mutation	Childhood	Nonprogressive chorea with early onset in childhood
Chorea-acanthocytosis	AR	*VPS13A*	Point mutation	20–30	Similar to HD, while more orofacial involvement
Wilson's disease	AR	*ATP7B*	Point mutation/insertion/deletion	3–80	Most commonly present with parkinsonism and dystonia, only 9% with chorea

AD autosomal dominant, *AR* autosomal recessive, *DRPLA* dentatorubral-pallidoluysian atrophy, *HD* Huntington's disease, *HDL* Huntington's disease-like

prevalent neurological symptom after cerebellar ataxia, followed by psychiatric symptoms, pyramidal signs, involuntary movements, parkinsonism, and epilepsy [76]. In this case, the patient was presented with the top four features of SCA17 (ataxia, dementia, psychiatric symptoms, and pyramidal signs), while involuntary movements, parkinsonism, and epilepsy were absent. We speculated that the absence of HDL symptoms might be due to the relatively short disease duration. Thus, the patient should be kept on following up.

Previous neurohistopathological findings revealed that neuronal loss of SCA17 might involve the cerebral cortex, subthalamic nucleus, ventral thalamic nuclei, cerebellar Purkinje cell layer and dentate nucleus, substantia nigra, and superior and inferior olive [77]. Therefore, brain MRI findings vary greatly in SCA17. Mild to moderate atrophy of local or global cerebellum might be presented in patients with disease duration no more than 3 years [78, 79]. The atrophy might spread to the cerebrum and brainstem later in the disease course.

In brief, SCA17 is a rare neurodegenerative disorder and shows a series of nonspecific cerebellar symptoms. It might be confused with HD when symptoms mimic which. Therefore, gene screenings of HDLs, especially SCA17, are highly recommended when the gene test for HD is negative.

1.8 Dentatorubral-Pallidoluysian Atrophy (DRPLA)

A 51-Year-Old Male Presented with an Unsteady Gait and Slurred Speech

Clinical Presentations

The patient was a 51-year-old male. He manifested as an unsteady gait and slurred speech at age 43 that gradually progressed. He developed involuntary twisting movement of four extremities and psychiatric symptoms such as delusions and hallucinations and had self-injurious behavior sometimes at age 46. After that, he gradually suffered memory loss and could not find a way back home and recognize family members when he was admitted to our hospital at age 51. There were four male and female family members in three consecutive generations that had similar symptoms (Fig. 1.22). Other medical history was unremarkable. Neurologic examinations showed that power of memory, orientation, and calculation decreased dramatically. Athetoid movements were found in four extremities. Cranial nerves were negative except for horizontal nystagmus. Muscle strength, muscle tone, and deep tendon reflexes were normal, but bilateral Babinski signs were positive. Finger-nose and heel-knee-shin tests were damaged. Sensory system was unimpaired and meningeal irritation sign was negative. The blood routine examination was normal. Brainstem and cerebellum were severe atrophic in magnetic resonance imaging (MRI) (Fig. 1.23).

The proband's nephew (III$_7$) was 15 years old. He gradually developed unsteady gait, slurred speech, and deteriorated cognition when he was 11 years old. He suffered from generalized tonic-clonic convulsions several times at the beginning of 12 years old. Neurologic examinations were not allowed.

Primary Diagnosis

The family presented with progressive cerebellar ataxia, nystagmus, and positive bilateral Babinski signs. These symptoms, signs, and atrophic brainstem and cerebellum in MRI indicated the involvement of the cerebellum, brainstem, and pyramidal system. Plus to the autosomal dominant

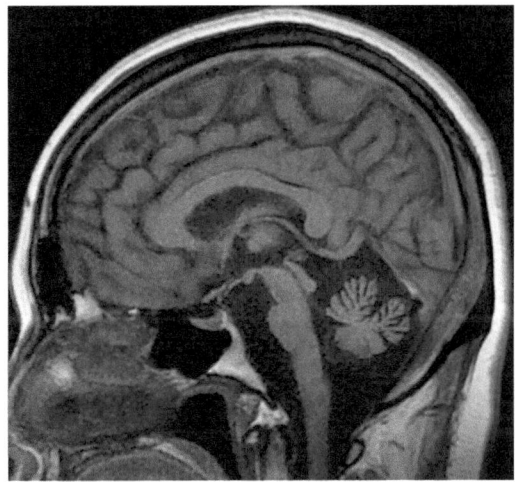

Fig. 1.23 Brain magnetic resonance imaging (MRI) of the patient. Sagittal T1-weighted image showed severe atrophy of the brainstem and cerebellum

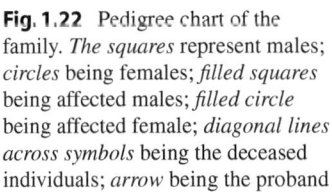

Fig. 1.22 Pedigree chart of the family. *The squares* represent males; *circles* being females; *filled squares* being affected males; *filled circle* being affected female; *diagonal lines across symbols* being the deceased individuals; *arrow* being the proband

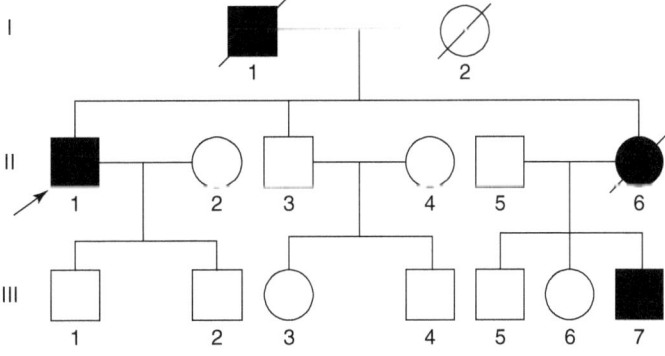

inheritance, the diagnosis of spinocerebellar ataxia (SCA) could be made. And since the symptoms also included dementia, psychiatric abnormity, epilepsy, and choreoathetosis, the diagnosis of dentatorubral-pallidoluysian atrophy (DRPLA) should be considered.

For the differential diagnosis, Huntington's disease (HD) was the major disease needed to excluded, since HD could also present with choreoathetosis, dementia, and psychiatric disturbance. Ataxia was the key symptom for differentiating DRPLA from HD. Some cases of DRPLA might exhibit pure cerebellar symptoms without dementia, choreoathetosis, or behavior changes. These cases need to be distinguished from other common SCA subtypes. Therefore, gene analysis to *ATN1* which was the causing gene of DRPLA should be carried out to confirm the diagnosis.

Additional Tests or Key Results

The CAG repeat expansion located in exon 5 of *ATN1* was amplified via polymerase chain reaction (PCR), and the PCR product was electrophoresed and sequenced. II_1 and III_7 were identified to have an expanded allele and a normal allele via agarose gel electrophoresis analysis (Fig. 1.24).

After sequencing, CAG copy numbers of the expanded allele were 68 in the proband (II_1) (Fig. 1.25). This result further confirmed the diagnosis of DRPLA.

Discussion

DRPLA was a rare autosomal dominant neurodegenerative disease. The name of "DRPLA"

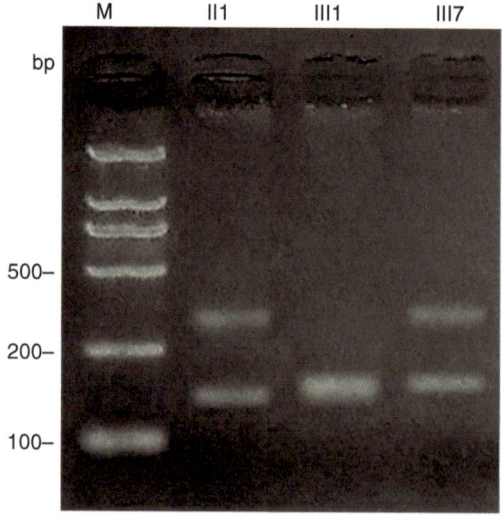

Fig. 1.24 The 2.5% agarose gel electrophoresis analysis of II_1, III_1, and III_7. M, DL2000

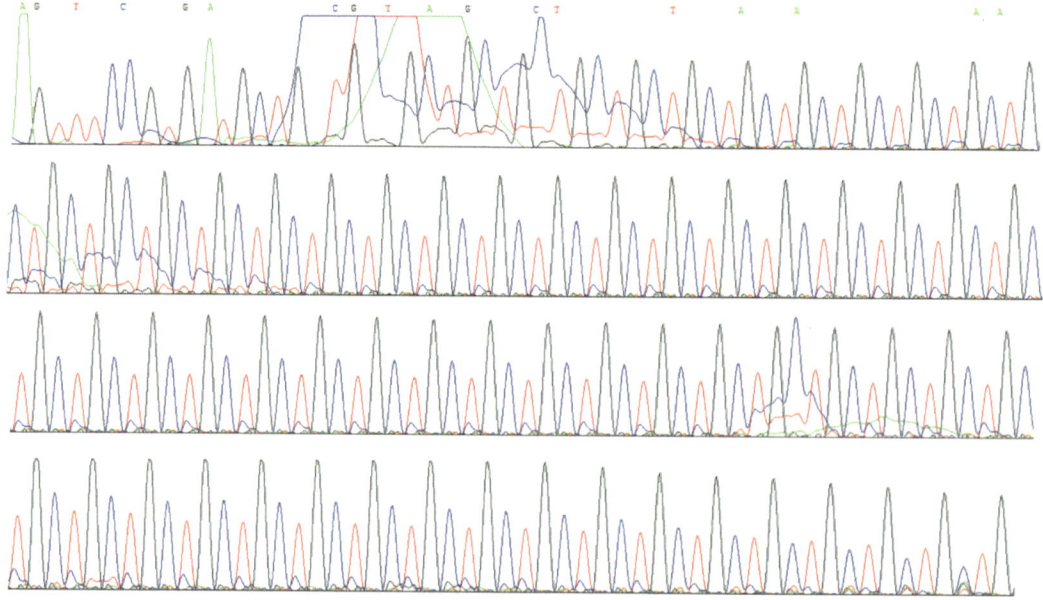

Fig. 1.25 Chromatogram shown in reverse sequence. II_1 harbored an expanded allele with 68 CAG repeats

was first described in a case with severe neuronal loss, particularly involving the dentatorubral and pallidoluysian systems in 1958 [80]. DRPLA was also named as Naito-Oyanagi disease in Japan, since Naito and Oyanagi summarized phenotypic characteristics of the disease in 1982 [81]. A large African-American family from the Haw River region in North Carolina presented with syndromes of ataxia, chorea, dementia, and seizures and was found to harbor CAG expanded mutation in *ATN1*. Therefore, DRPLA in this family was also referred to as Haw River syndrome [82]. Although DRPLA has been reported in several regions, including European and North and South American, most reported DRPLA cases are mainly from Japan. The prevalence of DRPLA was estimated at 0.48:100,000 based on the nationwide study in Japan [83]. DRPLA was caused by a CAG repeat expansion existing in exon 5 of the *ATN1* gene on chromosome12p13 [84]. The numbers of CAG repeats are 6–35 in normal individuals while 38–93 in DRPLA patients and inversely correlated with onset age. Since there were some similarities in clinical manifestations and hereditary mode between DRPLA and common

subtypes of SCA, DRPLA was regarded widely as one subtype of SCA.

DPRLA could manifest as various combinations of cerebellar ataxia, choreoathetosis, myoclonus, epilepsy, dementia, and psychiatric symptoms. The clinical manifestations were distinct depending on onset age. Cases with onset before age 20 years (early onset) usually presented with progressive ataxia, intellectual deterioration, progressive myoclonus epilepsy (PME), seizures, and myoclonus. Various forms of generalized seizures such as tonic, atonic, clonic, or tonic-clonic seizures were also observed. And the core features of cases with onset after age 20 years (adult onset) were including cerebellar ataxia, choreoathetosis, dementia, and psychiatric disturbance. The frequency of seizures decreased in patients with onset after the age of 20 and became very low after the age of 40 [85].

Similar to common SCA subtypes, there is no specific treatment for DRPLA. The principle of therapy for DRPLA is mainly symptomatic. Antiepileptic drugs, dopamine-blocking or depleting agents, and psychotropic medications could be chosen for seizures, movement disorders, and psychiatric problems, respectively.

1.9   Gerstmann-Straussler-Scheinker (GSS)

A 59-Year-Old Woman with Progressive Gait Unsteadiness

Clinical Presentations

A 59-year-old woman had a 4-year history of severe gait unsteadiness. She first noticed that she had difficulty maintaining balance while walking at age of 55. Since then, she underwent a gradual progression of gait difficulties. One year later, she exhibited a mild dysarthria but still had a relatively unimpaired swallowing ability. Meanwhile, she also had other problems including urinary incontinence and decreased libido. Three years after symptom onset, her medical condition deteriorated rapidly. Her personality changed a lot over the past three years. She became more irritable, grumpy, and was prone to tear. Her cognitive ability was impaired as well, which evaluated by Mini-Mental State Examination (MMSE) with a decreased score of 21/30. She was soon bedridden and received palliative care at home. She died at age 59 due to the respiratory and heart failure.

Past medical history was unremarkable. She had a long-standing history of cigarette habits. The similar symptoms were also observed in her other family members (Fig. 1.26). In her family, there were a total of six affected individuals. Her older brother (III-2) started the disease with mild

gait unsteadiness at the age of 48 and didn't exhibit any cognitive problem so far. Her cousin (III-10) exhibited gait difficulty at age of 45 and developed blurred speech and dysphagia at 50 years old. The other affected members (I-2, II-2, II-5) in this family experienced the similar symptoms with a relatively rapid disease progression. All of them died 3 or 4 years after symptom onset. No cognitive problem was documented in their medical records.

Upon neurological examination, one and a half years after onset, she had mild limited extraocular movements for upward gaze. The muscle strength was reduced in her four limbs, with strength 3/5 in lower limbs and 4/5 in upper limbs. Tendon reflexes were symmetrically decreased in both arms, but dramatically increased in both legs. Bilateral pathological signs were positive. Both finger-to-nose and heel-to-shin testings were positive. Gait testing revealed disequilibrium on standing and Romberg's test was also positive. Her sensory was not impaired.

There were no specific clinical findings on routine blood tests. Serum vitamin B12 and folic acid levels were normal. Routine cytological and biochemical examination of CSF disclosed unremarkable findings. The brain MRI revealed obvious cerebellar atrophy. MRI of thoracic and lumbar spinal showed a significant disc prolapse at T5–L1 level. There were no abnormal findings on electroencephalography

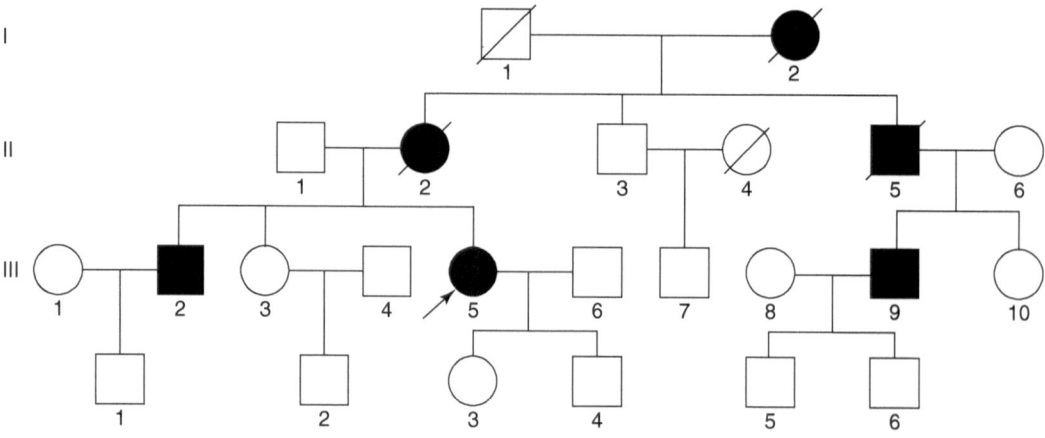

Fig. 1.26 Pedigree of the patient. *The squares* represent males; *circles* being females; *black symbols* being the affected individuals; *diagonal lines across symbols* being the deceased individuals; *arrow* being the proband

(EEG). Electromyography (EMG) revealed mild chronic neurogenic changes, which predominantly involved the right upper limb muscles innervated by cervical nerve roots (C7–C8) and the right lower limb muscles innervated by L5–S1 nerve root.

Primary Diagnosis

In this case, progressive gait unsteadiness, characterized later as ataxia, was the main symptom. The signs of ataxia also indicated dysfunction of cerebella. The cognitive disturbance developed in late stage accounts for the deficits of cerebral cortex. The observed pyramid signs suggested the impairment of the upper motor neuron. In addition, urinary incontinence and decreased libido highly suggested the involvement of autonomic nervous system. Therefore, primary anatomic locations included cerebella, cerebral, cortex, pyramidal, and autonomic nervous system. In present case, a clinical picture of gradual onset and slowly progressive course was obviously observed. This disease is obviously clustered within the family and inherited as an autosomal dominant pattern.

Ataxia was the most prominent feature of the patient over the entire course of the disease. Cognitive deficits developed relatively late when compared to ataxia. If dementia was the accompanied consequence of ataxia, autosomal dominant cerebellar ataxia (ADCA) should be considered as the most likely diagnosis. It is because that cognitive impairment can be commonly observed in some subtypes of ADCA, such as SCA2, SCA7, SCA15, and SCA17. Otherwise, if dementia occurred as an independent symptom, clinical suspicion of the diseases that influence both cerebella and cerebral cortex was needed. Genetic Creutzfeldt-Jakob disease (CJD) was the one of possible diagnosis that needs to be considered. Moreover, mitochondrial disease should also be differentiated because it often causes the dysfunction of multiple systems. Firstly, mitochondria disease appears to affect individuals with a relatively early age. Secondly, mitochondria disease causes not only the damage of brain and skeletal muscles but also other system of the body including the eye, cardiac, liver,

and endocrine and respiratory systems. Finally, mitochondria diseases are due to the mutation of genes encoded by mitochondrial DNA, following a maternal inheritance. The clinical feature of the present case didn't support the above characters of mitochondria disease, and thus, mitochondria disease can be excluded. Therefore, the genetic testing is required to help establish the correct diagnosis.

Additional Tests or Key Results

Nucleotide repeat expansion responsible for common subtypes of SCA, including SCA1, SCA2, SCA3, SCA6, SCA12, and SCA17, was tested. All repeats were confirmed in normal range. Through further targeted sequencing by combining the genes that cause ADCA through non-repeat mutations and several common dementia-related genes in a custom panel, the patient was finally detected with a known mutation (p.P102L) in *PRNP* gene. The mutation was further certificated through Sanger sequencing in his other affected family members (Fig. 1.27).

Discussion

Gerstmann-Sträussler-Scheinker (GSS) disease is an autosomal dominant inherited neurodegenerative disease, characterized by progressive cerebellar ataxia, dementia, parkinsonism, and pyramidal signs. It is a rare disease with an incidence rate estimated at 1 and 100 per 100 million [86]. The typical pathologic feature is an abnormal forma-

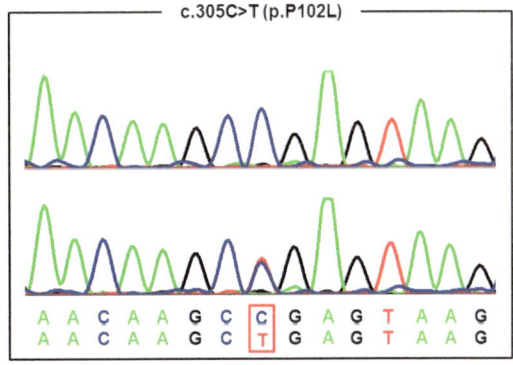

Fig. 1.27 Chromatogram of c.305C>T (p.P102L) mutation in *PRNP*. The upper panel is normal sequence, whereas the lower panel is heterozygous mutated sequence of the patient

tion of multiple amyloid plaques aggregated from prion protein (PRNP) [87]. The onset of GSS usually occurs between ages of 40 and 70, and the disease duration ranges from 1 to 10 years [88].

GSS is caused by the mutation in the prion protein (PRNP) gene, which is the only causative gene identified so far and recognized also as the culprit for the other two familial forms of prion diseases, including familial fatal insomnia and genetic Creutzfeldt-Jakob disease (CJD). More than 40 mutations in *PRNP* gene have been identified so far, and 15 of them (P84S, P102L, P105L, A117V, G131V, Y145X, V176G, H187R, F198S, D202G, E211D, Q212P, Q217A, Y218N, and M232T) are documented to be associated with GSS [89–92]. Of these mutations, P102L is the most common mutation reported in GSS cases worldwide.

Previous reports have indicated that a wide range of phenotype could be led by P102L mutation. The majority of patients carrying this mutation usually have a classic onset of midlife cerebellar ataxia, but there are still several cases reported previously with early-onset dementia [93, 94]. The present case displayed a typical clinical feature of early-onset ataxia and late development of dementia. Although many researchers attempt to establish the correlation between the phenotypic variation and genetic polymorphism at codons 129 or 219 of the PRNP gene, it turns out to be controversial.

Patients with GSS usually have symptoms similar to these patients being affected by SCA. It's difficult for clinicians to distinguish between GSS and SCA, especially in the early stage. In addition, the dominant inheritance pattern could further consolidate the clinical suspicion of ADCA. Here we excluded the abnormal repeat expansion of common subtypes of SCAs using the direct sequencing, which couldn't be done by next-generation sequencing. Through targeted sequencing, we identified a known mutation in this family.

Since an effective treatment of GSS is unavailable so far, early diagnosis and subsequent clinical cares of the patient are critical. We propose that the PRNP analysis should be applied to those patients with cerebellar ataxia in a dominant pattern, no matter whether they have cognitive problems.

1.10 Ataxia with Oculomotor Apraxia Type 2 (AOA2)

A 25-Year-Old Woman with Gait Unsteadiness and Tremble

Clinical Presentations

A 25-year-old woman with gait instability and tremble was referred to Neurology Department for workup. The gait unsteadiness, which had slowly progressed for 5 years, was observed by the patient and her families as the primary sign at the age of 20 years. After 1 year, her walk disability got worse, especially in the darkness. After 2 years of age at onset, she developed trunk and hand tremble with purposeful movements. Moreover, slurred speech and diplopia were seen. When she was assessed in our hospital, she showed conspicuous gait instability, poetry-like language, and tremble. It was impossible that she walked independently without support and stayed standing with feet together. Sensory symptoms, cognitive changes, or cardiorespiratory symptoms were absent.

There were normal mental and motor development histories for the patient. The family history disclosed the similar symptoms of gait unsteadiness and tremble in her sister, who had an onset at 16 years old. The parents and brother were away from the gait instability (Fig. 1.28). No other positive family history was reported, including hypertension, diabetes mellitus, or cardiomyopathy.

The normal vital signs and mentality status were revealed on examination. Neurologic examination

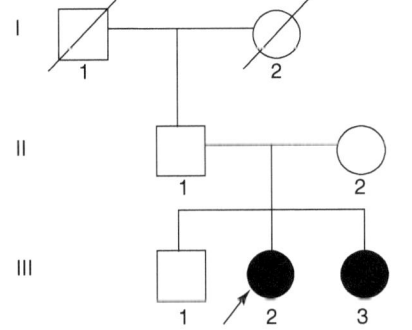

Fig. 1.28 Pedigree of the patient. *The squares* represent males; *circles* being females; *black symbols* being affected individuals; *diagonal lines across symbols* being the deceased individuals; *arrow* being the proband

demonstrated continuingly overt horizontal and vertical gaze-evoked nystagmus. Hand deformities, pes cavus, and moderate amyotrophy in the distal lower extremities were identified. However, vibratory and position senses were well preserved and muscle tone and strength were normal. Deep tendon reflexes were decreased in the upper limbs and disappeared in lower limbs. Furthermore, a weak Babinski sign in the right side was seen. Finger-nose test and heel-knee tests were performed with dysmetria. The administration of SARA (Scale for the Assessment and Rating of Ataxia), ICARS (International Cooperative Ataxia Rating Scale), and MMSE (Mini-Mental State Examination) yielded scores of 14.5/40, 38/100, and 28/30, respectively. The laboratory evaluation revealed normal creatine kinase, ferritin, vitamin B12, ceruloplasmin, IgG, blood glucose, and thyroid-stimulating hormone. The low-density lipoprotein of 1.68 nmol/L and albumin of 32.3 g/L were slightly decreased (normal LDL 2.1 ~ 3.1 nmol/L, normal albumin 35.0 ~ 52.0 g/L). Brain MRI at onset was unremarkable. Nevertheless, 3 years after age at onset, brain MRI showed for the first time the mild cerebellar atrophy. In addition, the EMG with nerve conduction studies demonstrated a multiple sensorimotor neuropathy with decreased amplitude and conduction velocity in median, tibial, sural, as well as peroneal nerves. Meanwhile, tibial anterior and femoral medial muscle both had neurogenic injury.

Primary Diagnosis

The patient was characterized by gait ataxia and tremor. On examination, there were poem-like language, nystagmus, hand deformities, pes cavus, amyotrophy in the lower extremities, absent deep tendon reflexes, positive finger-nose test and heel-knee test, as well as a weak Babinski sign in the right side. Additionally, the brain MRI displayed mild cerebellar atrophy, and the EMG with nerve conduction studies demonstrated a multiple sensorimotor neuropathy. Thus, in this patient, the disease can localize to cerebellum, peripheral nerves, and suspectable pyramidal tract. Besides, the 5-year and slowly progressive course of her symptoms is more suggestive of an inherited disease than an acquired etiology. Furthermore, the history of gait ataxia with tremor in the sister but absent in parents indicates that it is a kind of autosomal recessive cerebellar ataxia (ARCA). Unfortunately, the differential diagnosis for ARCA with neuropathy is broad.

Additional Tests or Key Results

In this patient, the normal blood glucose and negative histories of diabetes mellitus as well as cardiomyopathy essentially point away from Friedreich's ataxia [95]. In order to further exclude Friedreich's ataxia, the patient was tested for the GAA dynamic repeat expansion in frataxin (FXN) gene with negative result.

Up to now, more than 30 causative genes have been identified in ARCA. Moreover, ARCA is highly clinically heterogeneous. It is a giant challenge to decide which gene should be screened merely depending on the patients' clinical manifestations. Therefore, targeted next-generation sequencing (NGS) was applied to screen the patient for ARCA causative genes. A panel with 39 ARCA causative genes was designed to identify the potential mutations (Table 1.2). Consequently, compound heterozygous mutations c.4660T>G (p.C1554G)/c.3190G>T (p.E1064X) in exon 10 of *SETX* were detected, not previously reported (Fig. 1.29), which were further confirmed by Sanger sequencing. Then, both the affected sister and unaffected parents underwent the sequencing corresponding to the identified mutations. Of course, sister were the same compound heterozygous mutations, mother was heterozygous p.C1554G mutation and the father p.E1064X mutation, respectively. The p. C1554G and p.E1064X mutations located in relatively conservative region of senataxin were both nonsense mutations and produced damaging impact on senataxin predicted by PolyPhen-2, SIFT, and MutationTaster. Besides, the novel mutations were absent in 500 healthy controls of matched ethnic origin. These evidences supported the pathogenicity of the novel mutations.

Following the concern for *SETX*, the causative gene of ataxia with oculomotor apraxia type 2 (AOA2), we carried out the evaluation of serum alpha-fetoprotein (AFP) and brain MRI in this patient and her affected sister. Strikingly, the level of serum AFP was both severely increased (81.8 ng/mL in the patient,

Table 1.2 List of genes responsible for ARCA

Number	Disease	Gene symbol
1	AOA1	APTX
2	AOA2	SETX
3	AOA3	PIK3R5
4	SCAN1	TDP1
5	SCAR5	ZNF592
6	SCAR7	TPP1
7	SCAR8	SYNE1
8	SCAR9	ADCK3
9	SCAR10	ANO10
10	SCAR11	SYT14
11	SCAR12	WWOX
12	SCAR13	GRM1
13	SCAR14	SPTBN2
14	SCAR15	KIAA0226
15	SCAR16	STUB1
16	AT	ATM
17	CTX	CYP27A1
18	PACA	PTF1A
19	NA	AMACR
20	Refsum disease	PHYH
21	Refsum disease	PEX7
22	BNHS	PNPLA6
23	MSS	SIL1
24	BVVLS1	SLC52A3
25	BVVSL2	SLC52A2
26	AXED	TTPA
27	WFS	WFS1
28	PHARC	ABHD12
29	ICRD	ACO2
30	ATCAY	ATCAY
31	CAMRQ1	VLDLR
32	CAMRQ2	WDR81
33	CAMRQ3	CA8
34	CAMRQ4	ATP8A2
35	LKPAT	CLCN2
36	AXPC1	FLVCR1
37	SESAME	KCNJ10
38	PTBHS	LAMA1
39	SANDO	POLG

ARCA autosomal recessive cerebellar ataxias

40.3 ng/mL in the sister, normal range < 20 ng/mL). Meanwhile, conspicuous cerebellar atrophy predominantly in vermis and hemispheres was seen on the brain MRI of the two individuals (Fig. 1.30). In the ARCA, elevated AFP can

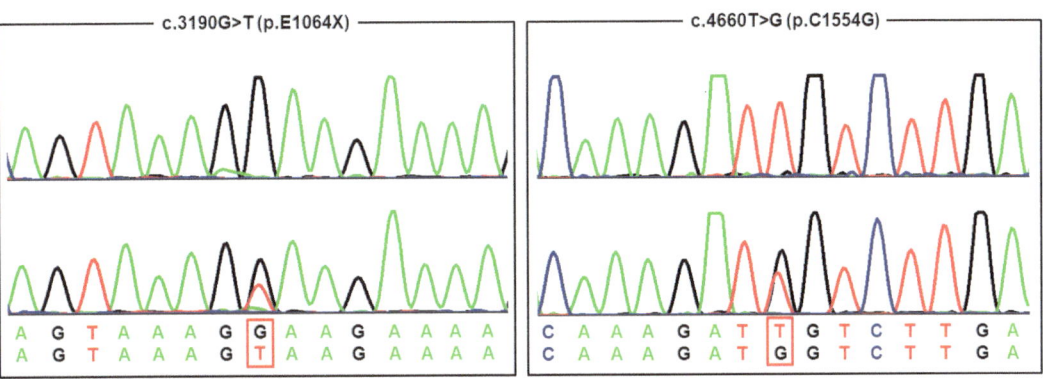

Fig. 1.29 Chromatogram of c.3190G>T mutation (**a**) and c.4660T>G mutation (**b**) within *SETX*. The upper row portrays the reference sequence. The lower panel depicts heterozygous mutated sequence

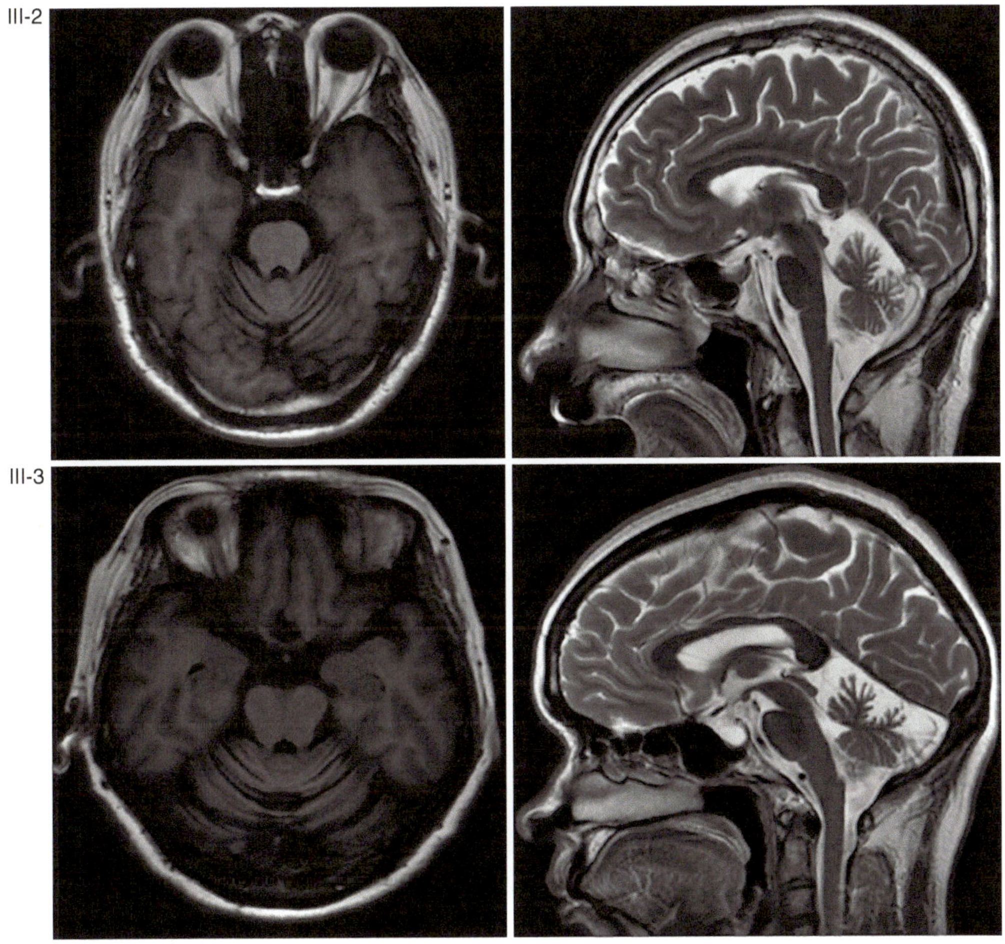

Fig. 1.30 Brain magnetic resonance imaging of the proband III-2 and the patient III-3. *Left*: axial T1-weighted image presenting atrophy of the cerebellar vermis. *Right*: midline sagittal T2-weighted image indicating cerebellar atrophy, particularly obvious in the vermis and hemispheres, with expansion of the fourth ventricle

appear in ataxia telangiectasia (AT) and AOA2, not in ataxia-telangiectasia-like disease (ATLD) or ataxia with oculomotor apraxia type 1 (AOA1) [96–100]. Unlike AOA2, AT is related to conjunctival telangiectasias, immunodeficiency, and earlier onset usually before 5 years of age [101, 102]. Accordingly, evidence mentioned above validates the diagnosis of AOA2.

Discussion

AOA2, one subtype of ARCA, was demonstrated as the second most frequent ARCA following Friedreich's ataxia [103]. The clinical presentation of AOA2 is highly heterogeneous, which is mainly relevant for juvenile-adolescent-onset cerebellar ataxia usually between 10 and 22 years of age, oculomotor apraxia, sensorimotor neuropathy, noted cerebellar atrophy on brain MRI, and increased serum level of AFP [104–108]. Oculomotor apraxia was defined as the inability to develop conative horizontal saccades with preserved reflex eye movements [109]. Although oculomotor apraxia is included in the disease acronym and occurred in 51% of the AOA2 cases previously reported, it is not a consistent characteristic [96, 103, 109–113] and also absent in this patient. This demonstrated that oculomotor apraxia might not be the primary factor for the diagnosis of AOA2. Alternatively, the case has not developed oculomotor apraxia yet for the early course of the disease.

It is known that AOA2 is caused by SETX mutations. AOA2 is a kind of rare neurodegenerative disease and has much phenotypic overlap with other ataxias, easily leading the misdiagnosis in clinical practice. Although the pathophysiology of elevated AFP level remains undefined, it seems to be a favorable biomarker in AOA2 diagnosis. Therefore, the AFP level should be examined in individuals with a recessive family history, onset of cerebellar ataxia in earlier adulthood, oculomotor impairment and peripheral neuropathy. In case of an elevated AFP level, the diagnosis of AOA2 should be considered systematically and gene detection is powerful for the final definite diagnosis.

To this day, no causal therapy of an underlying genetic defect in AOA2 is available. The treatment therefore remains exclusively symptomatic and focuses on the main symptoms. Cerebellar ataxia can benefit from buspirone. The citicoline and Coenzyme Q10 can improve the metabolism of brain tissue and promote the recovery of neural function. Furthermore, the common strategy for treating cerebellar ataxia is regular physiotherapy.

References

1. Yeh TH, Lu CS, Chou YH, Chong CC, Wu T, Han NH, Chen RS. Autonomic dysfunction in Machado-Joseph disease. Arch Neurol. 2005;62(4):630–636.
2. Pradhan C, Yashavantha BS, Pal PK, Sathyaprabha TN. Spinocerebellar ataxias type 1, 2 and 3: a study of heart rate variability. Acta Neurol Scand. 2008; 117(5):337–342.
3. Lin IS, Wu RM, Lee-Chen GJ, Shan DE, Gwinn-Hardy K. The SCA17 phenotype can include features of MSA-C, PSP and cognitive impairment. Parkinsonism Relat Disord. 2007;13(4):246–249.
4. Durr A. Autosomal dominant cerebellar ataxias: polyglutamine expansions and beyond. Lancet Neurol. 2010;9(9):885–894.
5. Orr HT, Chung MY, Banfi S, Kwiatkowski TJ Jr, Servadio A, Beaudet AL, McCall AE, Duvick LA, Ranum LP, Zoghbi HY. Expansion of an unstable trinucleotide CAG repeat in spinocerebellar ataxia type 1. Nat Genet. 1993;4(3):221–226.
6. Schöls L, Bauer P, Schmidt T, Schulte T, Riess O. Autosomal dominant cerebellar ataxias: clinical features, genetics, and pathogenesis. Lancet Neurol. 2004;3(5):291–304.
7. Sánchez-Cruz G, Velázquez-Pérez L, Gómez-Peña L, Martínez-Góngora E, Castellano-Sánchez G, Santos-Falcón N. Dysautonomic features in patients with Cuban type 2 spinocerebellar ataxia. Rev Neurol. 2001;33(5):428–434.
8. Harding AE. Clinical features and classification of inherited ataxias. Adv Neurol. 1993;61:1–14.
9. Ilg W, Brötz D, Burkard S, Giese MA, Schöls L, Synofzik M. Long-term effects of coordinative training in degenerative cerebellar disease. Mov Disord. 2010;25(13):2239–2246.
10. Miyai I, Ito M, Hattori N, Mihara M, Hatakenaka M, Yagura H, Sobue G, Nishizawa M. Cerebellar ataxia rehabilitation trial in degenerative cerebellar diseases. Neurorehabil Neural Repair. 2012;26(5):515–522.
11. Dong Y, Sun YM, Liu ZJ, Ni W, Shi SS, Wu ZY. Chinese patients with Huntington's disease initially presenting with spinocerebellar ataxia. Clin Genet. 2013;83(4):380–383.
12. Harding AE. The clinical features and classification of the late onset autosomal dominant cerebellar

ataxias. A study of 11 families, including descendants of the 'the drew family of Walworth'. Brain. 1982; 105(Pt 1):1–28.

13. Pulst SM, Nechiporuk A, Nechiporuk T, Gispert S, Chen XN, Lopes-Cendes I, Pearlman S, Starkman S, Orozco-Diaz G, Lunkes A, DeJong P, Rouleau GA, Auburger G, Korenberg JR, Figueroa C, Sahba S. Moderate expansion of a normally biallelic trinucleotide repeat in spinocerebellar ataxia type 2. Nat Genet. 1996;14(3):269–276.

14. Cancel G, Dürr A, Didierjean O, Imbert G, Bürk K, Lezin A, Belal S, Benomar A, Abada-Bendib M, Vial C, Guimarães J, Chneiweiss H, Stevanin G, Yvert G, Abbas N, Saudou F, Lebre AS, Yahyaoui M, Hentati F, Vernant JC, Klockgether T, Mandel JL, Agid Y, Brice A. Molecular and clinical correlations in spinocerebellar ataxia 2: a study of 32 families. Hum Mol Genet. 1997;6(5):709–715.

15. Kraft S, Furtado S, Ranawaya R, Parboosingh J, Bleoo S, McElligott K, Bridge P, Spacey S, Das S, Suchowersky O. Adult onset spinocerebellar ataxia in a Canadian movement disorders clinic. Can J Neurol Sci. 2005;32(4):450–458.

16. Geschwind DH, Perlman S, Figueroa CP, Treiman LJ, Pulst SM. The prevalence and wide clinical spectrum of the spinocerebellar ataxia type 2 trinucleotide repeat in patients with autosomal dominant cerebellar ataxia. Am J Hum Genet. 1997;60(4):842–850.

17. Sasaki H, Fukazawa T, Wakisaka A, Hamada K, Hamada T, Koyama T, Tsuji S, Tashiro K. Central phenotype and related varieties of spinocerebellar ataxia 2 (SCA2): a clinical and genetic study with a pedigree in the Japanese. J Neurol Sci. 1996; 144(1–2):176–181.

18. Bhalsing KS, Sowmya V, Netravathi M, Jain S, Pal PK. Spinocerebellar ataxia (SCA) type 2 presenting with chorea. Parkinsonism Relat Disord. 2013; 19(12):1171–1172.

19. Underwood BR, Rubinsztein DC. Spinocerebellar ataxias caused by polyglutamine expansions: a review of therapeutic strategies. Cerebellum. 2008; 7(2):215–221.

20. Freund HJ1, Barnikol UB, Nolte D, Treuer H, Auburger G, Tass PA, Samii M, Sturm V. Subthalamic-thalamic DBS in a case with spinocerebellar ataxia type 2 and severe tremor-a unusual clinical benefit. Mov Disord. 2007;22(5):732–735.

21. Velázquez-Pérez L, Rodríguez-Labrada R, García-Rodríguez JC, Almaguer-Mederos LE, Cruz-Mariño T, Laffita-Mesa JM. A comprehensive review of spinocerebellar ataxia type 2 in Cuba. Cerebellum. 2011;10(2):184–198.

22. Gan SR, Shi SS, Wu JJ, Wang N, Zhao GX, Weng ST, Murong SX, Lu CZ, Wu ZY. High frequency of Machado-Joseph disease identified in southeastern Chinese kindreds with spinocerebellar ataxia. BMC Med Genet. 2010;11:47.

23. Kawaguchi Y, Okamoto T, Taniwaki M, Aizawa M, Inoue M, Katayama S, Kawakami H, Nakamura S, Nishimura M, Akiguchi I, et al. CAG expansions in a novel gene for Machado-Joseph disease at chromosome 14q32.1. Nat Genet. 1994;8(3):221–228.

24. Takiyama Y, Oyanagi S, Kawashima S, Sakamoto H, Saito K, Yoshida M, Tsuji S, Mizuno Y, Nishizawa M. A clinical and pathologic study of a large Japanese family with Machado-Joseph disease tightly linked to the DNA markers on chromosome 14q. Neurology. 1994;44(7):1302–1308.

25. Riess O, Rub U, Pastore A, Bauer P, Schols L. SCA3: neurological features, pathogenesis and animal models. Cerebellum. 2008;7(2):125–137.

26. Sakai T, Kawakami H. Machado-Joseph disease: a proposal of spastic paraplegic subtype. Neurology. 1996;46(3):846–847.

27. Gan SR, Zhao K, Wu ZY, Wang N, Murong SX. Chinese patients with Machado-Joseph disease presenting with complicated hereditary spastic paraplegia. Eur J Neurol. 2009;16(8):953–956.

28. Wang YG, Du J, Wang JL, Chen J, Chen C, Luo YY, Xiao ZQ, Jiang H, Yan XX, Xia K, Pan Q, Tang BS, Shen L. Six cases of SCA3/MJD patients that mimic hereditary spastic paraplegia in clinic. J Neurol Sci. 2009;285(1-2):121–124.

29. Fowler HL. Machado-Joseph-Azorean disease. A ten-year study. Arch Neurol. 1984;41(9):921–925.

30. Lin KP, Soong BW. Peripheral neuropathy of Machado-Joseph disease in Taiwan: a morphometric and genetic study. Eur Neurol. 2002;48(4):210–217.

31. Kinoshita A, Hayashi M, Oda M, Tanabe H. Clinicopathological study of the peripheral nervous system in Machado-Joseph disease. J Neurol Sci. 1995;130(1):48–58.

32. Kanda T, Isozaki E, Kato S, Tanabe H, Oda M. Type III Machado-Joseph disease in a Japanese family: a clinicopathological study with special reference to the peripheral nervous system. Clin Neuropathol. 1989;8(3):134–141.

33. Soong BW, Lin KP. An electrophysiologic and pathological study of peripheral nerves in individuals with Machado-Joseph disease. Zhonghua Yi Xue Za Zhi (Taipei). 1998;61(4):181–187.

34. Coutinho P, Guimaraes A, Pires MM, Scaravilli F. The peripheral neuropathy in Machado-Joseph disease. Acta Neuropathol. 1986;71(1–2):119–124.

35. Fujioka S, Sundal C, Wszolek ZK. Autosomal dominant cerebellar ataxia type III: a review of the phenotypic and genotypic characteristics. Orphanet J Rare Dis. 2013;8:14.

36. Zhuchenko O, Bailey J, Bonnen P, Ashizawa T, Stockton DW, Amos C, Dobyns WB, Subramony SH, Zoghbi HY, Lee CC. Autosomal dominant cerebellar ataxia (SCA6) associated with small polyglutamine expansions in the alpha 1A-voltage-dependent calcium channel. Nat Genet. 1997;15(1):62–69.

37. Gomez CM, Thompson RM, Gammack JT, Perlman SL, Dobyns WB, Truwit CL, Zee DS, Clark HB, Anderson JH. Spinocerebellar ataxia type 6: gaze-evoked and vertical nystagmus, Purkinje cell degeneration, and variable age of onset. Ann Neurol. 1997;42(6):933–950.

38. Stevanin G, Durr A, David G, Didierjean O, Cancel G, Rivaud S, Tourbah A, Warter JM, Agid Y, Brice A. Clinical and molecular features of spinocerebellar ataxia type 6. Neurology. 1997;49(5):1243–1246.

39. Maruyama H, Izumi Y, Morino H, Oda M, Toji H, Nakamura S, Kawakami H. Difference in disease-free survival curve and regional distribution according to subtype of spinocerebellar ataxia: a study of 1,286 Japanese patients. Am J Med Genet. 2002;114(5):578–583.

40. Ishikawa K, Tanaka H, Saito M, Ohkoshi N, Fujita T, Yoshizawa K, Ikeuchi T, Watanabe M, Hayashi A, Takiyama Y, Nishizawa M, Nakano I, Matsubayashi K, Miwa M, Shoji S, Kanazawa I, Tsuji S, Mizusawa H. Japanese families with autosomal dominant pure cerebellar ataxia map to chromosome 19p13.1-p13.2 and are strongly associated with mild CAG expansions in the spinocerebellar ataxia type 6 gene in chromosome 19p13.1. Am J Hum Genet. 1997;61(2):336–346.

41. Matsumura R, Futamura N, Fujimoto Y, Yanagimoto S, Horikawa H, Suzumura A, Takayanagi T. Spinocerebellar ataxia type 6. Molecular and clinical features of 35 Japanese patients including one homozygous for the CAG repeat expansion. Neurology. 1997;49(5):1238–1243.

42. Mariotti C, Gellera C, Grisoli M, Mineri R, Castucci A, Di Donato S. Pathogenic effect of an intermediate-size SCA-6 allele (CAG)(19) in a homozygous patient. Neurology. 2001;57(8):1502–1504.

43. Rub U, Schols L, Paulson H, Auburger G, Kermer P, Jen JC, Seidel K, Korf HW, Deller T. Clinical features, neurogenetics and neuropathology of the polyglutamine spinocerebellar ataxias type 1, 2, 3, 6 and 7. Prog Neurobiol. 2013;104:38–66.

44. Gierga K, Schelhaas HJ, Brunt ER, Seidel K, Scherzed W, Egensperger R, de Vos RA, den Dunnen W, Ippel PF, Petrasch-Parwez E, Deller T, Schols L, Rub U. Spinocerebellar ataxia type 6 (SCA6): neurodegeneration goes beyond the known brain predilection sites. Neuropathol Appl Neurobiol. 2009;35(5):515–527.

45. Yabe I, Sasaki H, Yamashita I, Takei A, Tashiro K. Clinical trial of acetazolamide in SCA6, with assessment using the ataxia rating scale and body stabilometry. Acta Neurol Scand. 2001;104(1):44–47.

46. Assadi M, Campellone JV, Janson CG, Veloski JJ, Schwartzman RJ, Leone P. Treatment of spinocerebellar ataxia with buspirone. J Neurol Sci. 2007;260(1–2):143–146.

47. Trouillas P, Xie J, Adeleine P, Michel D, Vighetto A, Honnorat J, Dumas R, Nighoghossian N, Laurent B. Buspirone, a 5-hydroxytryptamine1A agonist, is active in cerebellar ataxia. Results of a double-blind drug placebo study in patients with cerebellar cortical atrophy. Arch Neurol. 1997;54(6):749–752.

48. Takei A, Hamada S, Homma S, Hamada K, Tashiro K, Hamada T. Difference in the effects of tandospirone on ataxia in various types of spinocerebellar degeneration: an open-label study. Cerebellum. 2010;9(4):567–570.

49. Romano S, Coarelli G, Marcotulli C, Leonardi L, Piccolo F, Spadaro M, Frontali M, Ferraldeschi M, Vulpiani MC, Ponzelli F, Salvetti M, Orzi F, Petrucci A, Vanacore N, Casali C, Ristori G. Riluzole in patients with hereditary cerebellar ataxia: a randomised, double-blind, placebo-controlled trial. Lancet Neurol. 2015;14(10):985–991.

50. Vaclavik V, Borruat FX, Ambresin A, Munier FL. Novel maculopathy in patients with spinocerebellar ataxia type 1 autofluorescence findings and functional characteristics. JAMA Ophthalmol. 2013;131(4):536–538.

51. Rufa A, Dotti MT, Galli L, Orrico A, Sicurelli F, Federico A. Spinocerebellar ataxia type 2 (SCA2) associated with retinal pigmentary degeneration. Eur Neurol. 2002;47(2):128–129.

52. Isashiki Y, Kii Y, Ohba N, Nakagawa M. Retinopathy associated with Machado–Joseph disease (spinocerebellar ataxia 3) with CAG trinucleotide repeat expansion. Am J Ophthalmol. 2001;131(6):808–810.

53. Finsterer J. Inherited mitochondrial disorders. Adv Exp Med Biol. 2012;942:187–213.

54. Harding AE. Classification of the hereditary ataxias and paraplegias. Lancet. 1983;1(8334):1151–1155.

55. David G, Abbas N, Stevanin G, Dürr A, Yvert G, Cancel G, Weber C, Imbert G, Saudou F, Antoniou E, Drabkin H, Gemmill R, Giunti P, Benomar A, Wood N, Ruberg M, Agid Y, Mandel JL, Brice A. Cloning of the SCA7 gene reveals a highly unstable CAG repeat expansion. Nat Genet. 1997;17(1):65–70.

56. Michalik A, Martin JJ, Van Broeckhoven C. Spinocerebellar ataxia type 7 associated with pigmentary retinal dystrophy. Eur J Hum Genet. 2004;12(1):2–15.

57. Miller RC, Tewari A, Miller JA, Garbern J, Van Stavern GP. Neuroophthalmologic features of spinocerebellar ataxia type 7. J Neuroophthalmol. 2009;29(3):180–186.

58. Whitney A, Lim M, Kanabar D, Lin JP. Massive SCA7 expansion detected in a 7-month-old male with hypotonia, cardiomegaly, and renal compromise. Dev Med Child Neurol. 2007;49(2):140–143.

59. Gan SR, Ni W, Zhao GX, Wu ZY. Clinical and molecular analyses of a Chinese spinocerebellar ataxia type 7 family that includes infantile-onset cases. Neurol Asia. 2012;17(2):121–126.

60. Wang J, Shen L, Lei L, Xu Q, Zhou J, Liu Y, Guan W, Pan Q, Xia K, Tang B, Jiang H. Spinocerebellar ataxias in mainland China: an updated genetic analysis among a large cohort of familial and sporadic cases. Zhong Nan Da Xue Xue Bao Yi Xue Ban. 2011;36(6):482–489.

61. Fujigasaki H, Verma IC, Camuzat A, Margolis RL, Zander C, Lebre AS, Jamot L, Saxena R, Anand I, Holmes SE, Ross CA, Durr A, Brice A. SCA12 is a rare locus for autosomal dominant cerebellar ataxia: a study of an Indian family. Ann Neurol. 2001;49(1):117–121.

62. Holmes SE, O'Hearn EE, McInnis MG, Gorelick-Feldman DA, Kleiderlein JJ, Callahan C, Kwak NG,

Ingersoll-Ashworth RG, Sherr M, Sumner AJ, Sharp AH, Ananth U, Seltzer WK, Boss MA, Vieria-Saecker AM, Epplen JT, Riess O, Ross CA, Margolis RL. Expansion of a novel CAG trinucleotide repeat in the 5′ region of PPP2R2B is associated with SCA12. Nat Genet. 1999;23(4):391–392.

63. Srivastava AK, Choudhry S, Gopinath MS, Roy S, Tripathi M, Brahmachari SK, Jain S. Molecular and clinical correlation in five Indian families with spinocerebellar ataxia 12. Ann Neurol. 2001;50(6): 796–800.

64. Bahl S, Virdi K, Mittal U, Sachdeva MP, Kalla AK, Holmes SE, O'Hearn E, Margolis RL, Jain S, Srivastava AK, Mukerji M. Evidence of a common founder for SCA12 in the Indian population. Ann Hum Genet. 2005;69(Pt 5):528–534.

65. Zhao Y, Tan EK, Law HY, Yoon CS, Wong MC, Ng I. Prevalence and ethnic differences of autosomal-dominant cerebellar ataxia in Singapore. Clin Genet. 2002;62(6):478–481.

66. Brusco A, Cagnoli C, Franco A, Dragone E, Nardacchione A, Grosso E, Mortara P, Mutani R, Migone N, Orsi L. Analysis of SCA8 and SCA12 loci in 134 Italian ataxic patients negative for SCA1-3, 6 and 7 CAG expansions. J Neurol. 2002;249(7):923–929.

67. Xie QY, Liang XL, Li XH. Molecular genetics and its clinical application in the diagnosis of spinocerebellar ataxias. Zhonghua Yi Xue Yi Chuan Xue Za Zhi. 2005;22(1):71–73.

68. Li HT, Lei J, Ma JH, Yu J, Zhang XN. Gene mutation and clinical characteristics of a Chinese Uygur family with spinocerebellar ataxia type 12. Zhonghua Yi Xue Yi Chuan Xue Za Zhi. 2011;28(2):137–141.

69. O'Hearn E, Holmes SE, Calvert PC, Ross CA, Margolis RL. SCA-12: tremor with cerebellar and cortical atrophy is associated with a CAG repeat expansion. Neurology. 2001;56(3):299–303.

70. Koide R, Kobayashi S, Shimohata T, Ikeuchi T, Maruyama M, Saito M, Yamada M, Takahashi H, Tsuji S. A neurological disease caused by an expanded CAG trinucleotide repeat in the TATA-binding protein gene: a new polyglutamine disease? Hum Mol Genet. 1999;8(11):2047–2053.

71. Nakamura K, Jeong SY, Uchihara T, Anno M, Nagashima K, Nagashima T, Ikeda S, Tsuji S, Kanazawa I. SCA17, a novel autosomal dominant cerebellar ataxia caused by an expanded polyglutamine in TATA-binding protein. Hum Mol Genet. 2001;10(14):1441–1448.

72. van Roon-Mom WM, Reid SJ, Faull RL, Snell RG. TATA-binding protein in neurodegenerative disease. Neuroscience. 2005;133(4):863–872.

73. Gao R, Matsuura T, Coolbaugh M, Zuhlke C, Nakamura K, Rasmussen A, Siciliano MJ, Ashizawa T, Lin X. Instability of expanded CAG/CAA repeats in spinocerebellar ataxia type 17. Eur J Hum Genet. 2008;16(2):215–222.

74. Govert F, Schneider SA. Huntington's disease and Huntington's disease-like syndromes: an overview. Curr Opin Neurol. 2013;26(4):420–427.

75. Schneider SA, van de Warrenburg BP, Hughes TD, Davis M, Sweeney M, Wood N, Quinn NP, Bhatia KP. Phenotypic homogeneity of the Huntington disease-like presentation in a SCA17 family. Neurology. 2006;67(9):1701–1703.

76. Stevanin G, Brice A. Spinocerebellar ataxia 17 (SCA17) and Huntington's disease-like 4 (HDL4). Cerebellum. 2008;7(2):170–178.

77. Rolfs A, Koeppen AH, Bauer I, Bauer P, Buhlmann S, Topka H, Schols L, Riess O. Clinical features and neuropathology of autosomal dominant spinocerebellar ataxia (SCA17). Ann Neurol. 2003;54(3):367–375.

78. Zuhlke C, Hellenbroich Y, Dalski A, Kononowa N, Hagenah J, Vieregge P, Riess O, Klein C, Schwinger E. Different types of repeat expansion in the TATA-binding protein gene are associated with a new form of inherited ataxia. Eur J Hum Genet. 2001;9(3): 160–164.

79. Hagenah JM, Zuhlke C, Hellenbroich Y, Heide W, Klein C. Focal dystonia as a presenting sign of spinocerebellar ataxia 17. Mov Disord. 2004;19(2): 217–220.

80. Smith JK, Gonda VE, Malamud N. Unusual form of cerebellar ataxia: combined dentato-rubral and pallido-Luysian degeneration. Neurology. 1958;8: 205–209.

81. Naito H, Oyanagi S. Familial myoclonus epilepsy and choreoathetosis: hereditary dentatorubral-pallidoluysian atrophy. Neurology. 1982;32:798–807.

82. Burke JR, Ikeuchi T, Koide R, Tsuji S, Yamada M, Pericak-Vance MA, Vance JM. Dentatorubral-pallidoluysian atrophy and Haw River syndrome. Lancet. 1994;344:1711–1712.

83. Tsuji S, Onodera O, Goto J, Nishizawa M, Study Group on Ataxic Diseases. Sporadic ataxias in Japan—a population-based epidemiological study. Cerebellum. 2008;7:189–197.

84. Koide R, Ikeuchi T, Onodera O, Tanaka H, Igarashi S, Endo K, Takahashi H, Kondo R, Ishikawa A, Hayashi T, Saito M, Tomoda A, Miike T, Naito H, Ikuta F, Tsuji S. Unstable expansion of CAG repeat in hereditary dentatorubral-pallidoluysian atrophy (DRPLA). Nat Genet. 1994;6:9–13.

85. Tsuji S. Dentatorubral-pallidoluysian atrophy. Handb Clin Neurol. 2012;103:587–594.

86. Kovacs GG, Puopolo M, Ladogana A, Pocchiari M, Budka H, van Duijn C, Collins SJ, Boyd A, Giulivi A, Coulthart M, Delasnerie-Laupretre N, Brandel JP, Zerr I, Kretzschmar HA, de Pedro-Cuesta J, Calero-Lara M, Glatzel M, Aguzzi A, Bishop M, Knight R, Belay G, Will R, Mitrova E, Eurocjd. Genetic prion disease: the EUROCJD experience. Hum Genet. 2005;118(2):166–174.

87. Wadsworth JD, Joiner S, Linehan JM, Cooper S, Powell C, Mallinson G, Buckell J, Gowland I, Asante EA, Budka H, Brandner S, Collinge J. Phenotypic heterogeneity in inherited prion disease (P102L) is associated with differential propagation of protease-resistant wild-type and mutant prion protein. Brain. 2006;129(Pt 6):1557–1569.

88. Young K, Clark HB, Piccardo P, Dlouhy SR, Ghetti B. Gerstmann–Sträussler–scheinker disease with the PRNP P102L mutation and valine at codon 129. Mol Brain Res. 1997;44(1):147–150.

89. Liberski PP. Gerstmann-Sträussler-Scheinker disease[A]. In: Ahmad SI, editor. Neurodegenerative diseases. New York, NY: Springer US; 2012. p. 128–137.

90. Popova SN, Tarvainen I, Capellari S, Parchi P, Hannikainen P, Pirinen E, Haapasalo H, Alafuzoff I. Divergent clinical and neuropathological phenotype in a Gerstmann–Sträussler–Scheinker P102L family. Acta Neurol Scand. 2012;126(5):315–323.

91. Simpson M, Johanssen V, Boyd A, et al. UNusual clinical and molecular-pathological profile of gerstmann-sträussler-scheinker disease associated with a novel prnp mutation (v176g). JAMA Neurol. 2013;70(9):1180–1185.

92. Jones M, Odunsi S, du Plessis D, Vincent A, Bishop M, Head MW, Ironside JW, Gow D. Gerstmann-Sträussler-Scheinker disease: novel PRNP mutation and VGKC-complex antibodies. Neurology. 2014;82(23):2107–2111.

93. Giovagnoli AR, Di Fede G, Aresi A, Reati F, Rossi G, Tagliavini F. Atypical frontotemporal dementia as a new clinical phenotype of Gerstmann-Straussler-Scheinker disease with the PrP-P102L mutation. Description of a previously unreported Italian family. Neurol Sci. 2008;29(6):405–410.

94. Ferrer I, Carmona M, Blanco R, Recio MJR, San Segundo RM. Gerstmann-Sträussler-Scheinker PRNP P102L-129V mutation. Transl Neurosci. 2011;2(1): 23–32.

95. Durr A, Cossee M, Agid Y, Campuzano V, Mignard C, Penet C, Mandel JL, Brice A, Koenig M. Clinical and genetic abnormalities in patients with Friedreich's ataxia. N Engl J Med. 1996;335(16): 1169–1175.

96. Anheim M, Monga B, Fleury M, Charles P, Barbot C, Salih M, Delaunoy JP, Fritsch M, Arning L, Synofzik M, Schols L, Sequeiros J, Goizet C, Marelli C, Le Ber I, Koht J, Gazulla J, De Bleecker J, Mukhtar M, Drouot N, Ali-Pacha L, Benhassine T, Chbicheb M, M'Zahem A, Hamri A, Chabrol B, Pouget J, Murphy R, Watanabe M, Coutinho P, Tazir M, Durr A, Brice A, Tranchant C, Koenig M. Ataxia with oculomotor apraxia type 2: clinical, biological and genotype/phenotype correlation study of a cohort of 90 patients. Brain. 2009;132(Pt 10): 2688–2698.

97. Stray-Pedersen A, Borresen-Dale AL, Paus E, Lindman CR, Burgers T, Abrahamsen TG. Alpha fetoprotein is increasing with age in ataxia-telangiectasia. Eur J Paediatr Neurol. 2007;11(6): 375–380.

98. Anheim M, Fleury MC, Franques J, Moreira MC, Delaunoy JP, Stoppa-Lyonnet D, Koenig M, Tranchant C. Clinical and molecular findings of ataxia with oculomotor apraxia type 2 in 4 families. Arch Neurol. 2008;65(7):958–962.

99. Fernet M, Gribaa M, Salih MA, Seidahmed MZ, Hall J, Koenig M. Identification and functional consequences of a novel MRE11 mutation affecting 10 Saudi Arabian patients with the ataxia telangiectasia-like disorder. Hum Mol Genet. 2005;14(2):307–318.

100. Bohlega SA, Shinwari JM, Al Sharif LJ, Khalil DS, Alkhairallah TS, Al Tassan NA. Clinical and molecular characterization of ataxia with oculomotor apraxia patients in Saudi Arabia. BMC Med Genet. 2011;12:27.

101. Chun HH, Gatti RA. Ataxia-telangiectasia, an evolving phenotype. DNA Repair (Amst). 2004;3(8-9): 1187–1196.

102. Savitsky K, Bar-Shira A, Gilad S, Rotman G, Ziv Y, Vanagaite L, Tagle DA, Smith S, Uziel T, Sfez S, Ashkenazi M, Pecker I, Frydman M, Harnik R, Patanjali SR, Simmons A, Clines GA, Sartiel A, Gatti RA, Chessa L, Sanal O, Lavin MF, Jaspers NG, Taylor AM, Arlett CF, Miki T, Weissman SM, Lovett M, Collins FS, Shiloh Y. A single ataxia telangiectasia gene with a product similar to PI-3 kinase. Science. 1995;268(5218):1749–1753.

103. Le Ber I, Bouslam N, Rivaud-Pechoux S, Guimaraes J, Benomar A, Chamayou C, Goizet C, Moreira MC, Klur S, Yahyaoui M, Agid Y, Koenig M, Stevanin G, Brice A, Durr A. Frequency and phenotypic spectrum of ataxia with oculomotor apraxia 2: a clinical and genetic study in 18 patients. Brain. 2004;127(Pt 4):759–767.

104. Fogel BL, Perlman S. Clinical features and molecular genetics of autosomal recessive cerebellar ataxias. Lancet Neurol. 2007;6(3):245–257.

105. Le Ber I, Brice A, Durr A. New autosomal recessive cerebellar ataxias with oculomotor apraxia. Curr Neurol Neurosci Rep. 2005;5(5):411–417.

106. Criscuolo C, Chessa L, Di Giandomenico S, Mancini P, Sacca F, Grieco GS, Piane M, Barbieri F, De Michele G, Banfi S, Pierelli F, Rizzuto N, Santorelli FM, Gallosti L, Filla A, Casali C. Ataxia with oculomotor apraxia type 2: a clinical, pathologic, and genetic study. Neurology. 2006;66(8):1207–1210.

107. Chen YZ, Hashemi SH, Anderson SK, Huang Y, Moreira MC, Lynch DR, Glass IA, Chance PF, Bennett CL. Senataxin, the yeast Sen1p orthologue: characterization of a unique protein in which recessive mutations cause ataxia and dominant mutations cause motor neuron disease. Neurobiol Dis. 2006; 23(1):97–108.

108. Moreira MC, Klur S, Watanabe M, Nemeth AH, Le Ber I, Moniz JC, Tranchant C, Aubourg P, Tazir M, Schols L, Pandolfo M, Schulz JB, Pouget J, Calvas P, Shizuka-Ikeda M, Shoji M, Tanaka M, Izatt L, Shaw CE, M'Zahem A, Dunne E, Bomont P, Benhassine T, Bouslam N, Stevanin G, Brice A, Guimaraes J, Mendonca P, Barbot C, Coutinho P, Sequeiros J, Durr A, Warter JM, Koenig M. Senataxin, the ortholog of a yeast RNA helicase, is mutant in ataxia-ocular apraxia 2. Nat Genet. 2004;36(3):225–227.

109. Duquette A, Roddier K, McNabb-Baltar J, Gosselin I, St-Denis A, Dicaire MJ, Loisel L, Labuda D, Marchand L, Mathieu J, Bouchard JP, Brais B. Mutations in senataxin responsible for Quebec

cluster of ataxia with neuropathy. Ann Neurol. 2005; 57(3):408–414.

110. Nakamura K, Yoshida K, Makishita H, Kitamura E, Hashimoto S, Ikeda S. A novel nonsense mutation in a Japanese family with ataxia with oculomotor apraxia type 2 (AOA2). J Hum Genet. 2009;54(12): 746–748.

111. Vermeer S, Hoischen A, Meijer RP, Gilissen C, Neveling K, Wieskamp N, de Brouwer A, Koenig M, Anheim M, Assoum M, Drouot N, Todorovic S, Milic-Rasic V, Lochmuller H, Stevanin G, Goizet C, David A, Durr A, Brice A, Kremer B, van de Warrenburg BP, Schijvenaars MM, Heister A, Kwint M, Arts P, van der Wijst J, Veltman J, Kamsteeg EJ, Scheffer H, Knoers N. Targeted next-generation sequencing of a 12.5 Mb homozygous region reveals ANO10 mutations in patients with autosomal-recessive cerebellar ataxia. Am J Hum Genet. 2010;87(6):813–819.

112. Fogel BL, Perlman S. Novel mutations in the senataxin DNA/RNA helicase domain in ataxia with oculomotor apraxia 2. Neurology. 2006;67(11): 2083–2084.

113. Arning L, Schols L, Cin H, Souquet M, Epplen JT, Timmann D. Identification and characterisation of a large senataxin (SETX) gene duplication in ataxia with ocular apraxia type 2 (AOA2). Neurogenetics. 2008;9(4):295–299.

Epileptic Attack-Related Disorders

Qing-Qing Tao, Hong-Fu Li, and Sheng Chen

Abstract

Epileptic attacks can cause symptoms such as limb twitches, muscle spasms, loss of consciousness, and changes in behavior. There are many different kinds of epileptic attacks, which are usually described by their symptoms or by where in the brain they originate. Many causes can lead to epileptic attacks, including trauma, brain tumors, prenatal injury, medications, stroke, poisoning, heart attacks, alcoholism, and a variety of developmental and metabolic disorders. Genetics also play an important role. In this chapter, we will discuss several genetic epileptic attack-related disorders including MELAS, MERRF, TSC, and cherry-red spot myoclonus.

Keywords

Epileptic attacks • Genetics • MELAS • MERRF • TSC • Cherry-red spot myoclonus

Q.-Q. Tao (✉) • H.-F. Li • S. Chen
Department of Neurology and Research Center of
Neurology, Second Affiliated Hospital, Zhejiang
University School of Medicine, Hangzhou, China
e-mail: jasontaoqing@126.com

© Springer Nature Singapore Pte Ltd. 2017
Z.-Y. Wu (ed.), *Inherited Neurological Disorders*, DOI 10.1007/978-981-10-4196-9_2

2.1 Mitochondrial Encephalo-myopathy with Lactic Acidosis and Stroke-Like Episodes (MELAS)

A 20-Year-Old Girl with Transient Loss of Consciousness and Seizures

Clinical Presentations

A 20-year-old girl was admitted to our hospital with a chief complaint of transient loss of consciousness and seizures 1 week ago. The girl's father reported that she was on the floor, "frothing at the mouth" and stereotypic movements, with both arms flexed and both feet extended. The movements resolved within 60 s followed by malaise and dizziness for several hours. Past medical history revealed that she had an episode of fever and encephalopathy with left temporal and occipital cortex lobe swelling on brain CT 2 years before this admission. At that time, she was treated for suspected herpes encephalitis with acyclovir and corticosteroid. After 2 weeks' treatment, she made a nearly full recovery at discharge. Six months later, she presented abruptly headache and ablepsia and also made a full recovery after symptomatic treatments for 2 weeks. She was born after a full-term gestation and had normal growth and development. There was no family history of note (Fig. 2.1).

The neurological examinations showed a normal mental status and fluent speech. Examinations of the cranial nerves were unremarkable. Muscle strength was normal. She had a positive Babinski sign on the left. Tendon reflexes and sensory examinations were normal. Her neck was supple and Kernig's sign was negative.

The routine blood tests including full blood count, hematocrit, platelets, liver, kidney, and thyroid function disclosed unremarkable findings. Electrocardiogram (ECG) and heart, kidney, and abdominal Doppler ultrasound showed uninformative results. The appearances of abnormal electroencephalogram (EEG) were mainly slow wave. The brain MRI examination showed high signals in the right temporal and occipital

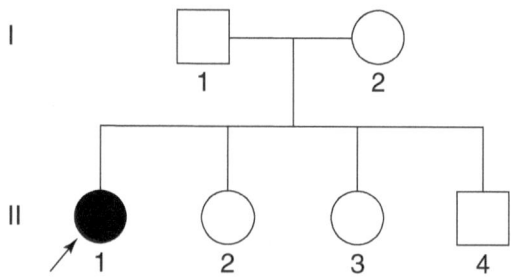

Fig. 2.1 Pedigree of the patient's family. *Circles* indicate females; *squares* indicate males; the *black symbols* indicate affected individuals; *diagonal lines across symbols* indicate deceased individuals; *arrows* indicate the probands

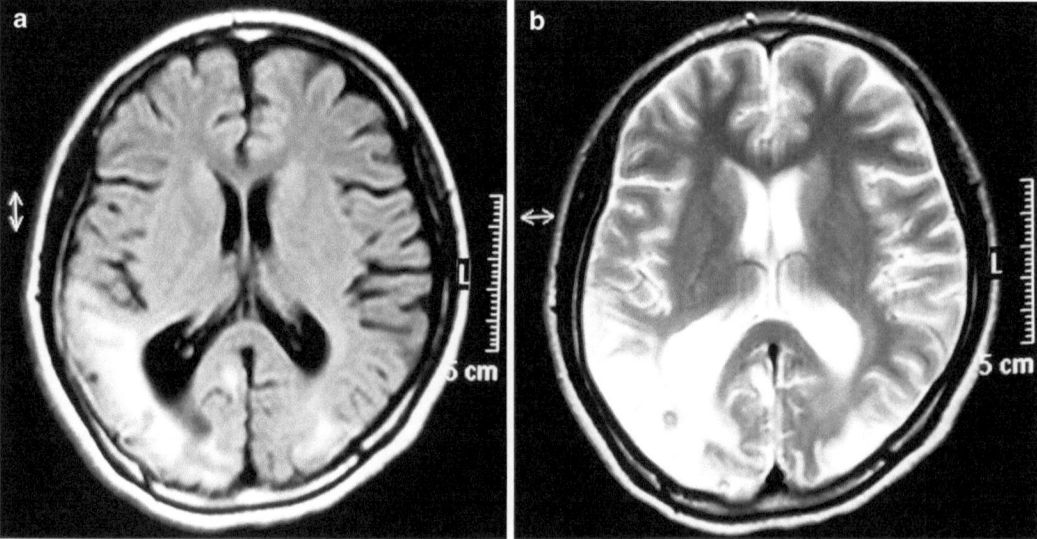

Fig. 2.2 Brain MRI showed high signals in the right temporal and occipital cortex as well as left occipital cortex on FLAIR (**a**) and T2-weighted images (**b**)

cortex as well as left occipital cortex on T2-weighted and fluid-attenuated inversion recovery (FLAIR) images (Fig. 2.2).

Primary Diagnosis

The clinical features of the patient including transient loss of consciousness, seizures, and positive Babinski sign hinted the involvement of cortex and pyramidal tract. Relatively young onset age, recurrent episodes, and neuroimaging manifestations implied that the possible diagnoses should include encephalitis, hereditary metabolic disease, and primary central nervous system (CNS) vasculitis. Additional tests including lumbar puncture, lactic acid test, and muscle biopsy should be performed to enhance the ability to make a diagnosis.

Additional Tests or Key Results

Intracranial pressure was normal, and routine cytological and biochemical examination of cerebrospinal fluid (CSF) disclosed unremarkable findings, which excluded the diagnosis of encephalitis. The clinical manifestations of CNS vasculitis are highly variable. Lack of specific noninvasive tests and materials for pathophysiologic investigation made it to be one of the most formidable diagnostic and therapeutic challenges for physicians [1]. The diagnosis of CNS vasculitis is secured by a positive brain biopsy. But as an invasive test, brain biopsy usually has low priority to perform. Basic lactic acid level from the blood was 2.9 mmol/L (reference range 0.7–

2.1 mmol/L), immediate blood lactic acid level after exercise was 9.6 mmol/L (reference range 0.7–2.1 mmol/L), and blood lactic acid level after 10 min rest was 5.1 mmol/L (reference range 0.7–2.1 mmol/L). The histological staining of the muscle tissue from the patient showed a basophilia ragged red fiber (RRF) by using hematoxylin and eosin (H&E) staining (Fig. 2.3a). RRF is also positive by modified Gomori trichrome (MGT) staining (Fig. 2.3b) and succinate dehydrogenase (SDH) staining (Fig. 2.3c). Investigations at this time included positive lactic acid test, and RRF found in muscle biopsy implied that mitochondrial diseases should be considered first. In retrospect, the patient's neuroimaging manifestations highly indicated that the probable diagnosis was mitochondrial myopathy, encephalopathy, lactic acidosis, and a stroke-like episode (MELAS). To confirm our hypothesis, we examined the most common mutation of MELAS and found positive mitochondrial mtDNA A3243G mutation thereby confirming the diagnosis (Fig. 2.4).

Discussion

MELAS is one of the most common mitochondrial disorders. It has variable clinical manifestations including motor weakness, epilepsy, recurrent headaches, hearing loss, myopathy, lactic academia, and short stature. m.3243A>G mutation is the most frequent mutation associated with MELAS [2].

The mtDNA is strictly inherited from the mother. The cells can contain varying propor-

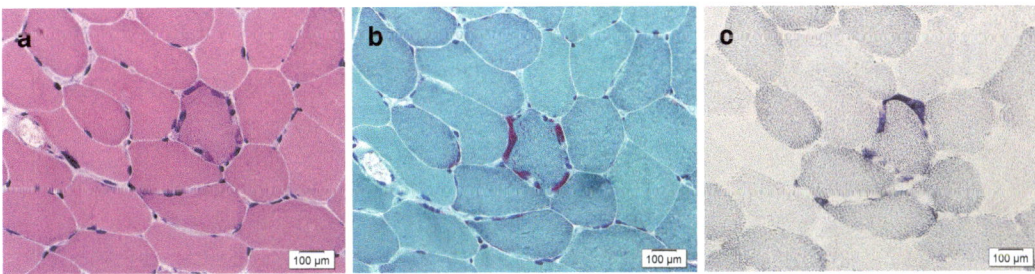

Fig. 2.3 Histologic staining of the muscle tissue from the patient shows a basophilia RRF by using hematoxylin and eosin (H&E) staining (**a**), MGT staining (**b**), and SDH staining (**c**)

Fig. 2.4 Chromatogram of m.3243A>G mutation detected in the patient

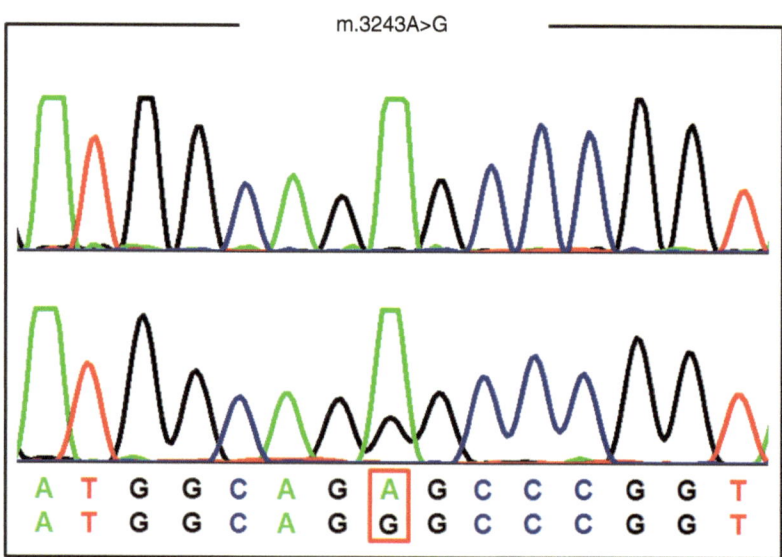

tions of mutated and wild-type mtDNA. They can usually tolerate a certain percentage of mutated mtDNA level. In most cases, clinical manifestation of the genetic defect occurs only when a threshold level is transcended. This phenomenon has been called the threshold effect. The abnormal mitochondria cannot generate enough energy to meet the needs of multiple organs leading to the multi-organ dysfunction.

In this case, the patient has a history of two stroke-like episodes. She made a nearly full recovery in both episodes. Stroke-like episodes are one of the major features of MELAS that demonstrate in over 80% of patients. These episodes demonstrate with partially reversible motor weakness, recurrent headaches, hearing impairment, cortical vision loss, aphasia, and seizures. The affected brain areas do not well correspond to classic vascular distribution, involving predominantly the temporal, parietal, and occipital lobes,

and also can affect subcortical white matter [3]. Epilepsy is also a common neurological manifestation occurring in over 71% of patients. Seizures can occur independently or as a result of a stroke-like episode. Other common manifestations include recurrent headaches, hearing impairment, myopathy, and lactic academia. Lactic academia in MELAS syndrome is due to the inability of abnormal mitochondria to generate sufficient oxidized glucose, leading to the accumulation of pyruvate and shunting of pyruvate to lactate. However, lactic academia can also occur in metabolic diseases and systemic disease.

There is no effective therapy for treating MELAS so far [4]. Symptomatic and supportive cares are the mainstay treatment for patients. Some compounds such as co-enzyme Q10, vitamin B1, vitamin B2, vitamin C, vitamin E, vitamin K, and alpha-lipoic acid may ameliorate symptoms for some patients.

2.2 Myoclonus Epilepsy Associated with Ragged Red Fibers (MERRF)

A 52-Year-Old Female Presented with Paroxysmal Right Upper Limb Tics

Clinical Presentations

A 52-year-old woman complained of paroxysmal right upper limb tics that have been ongoing for over 20 years came to our Neurology Clinic. The involuntary limb tics demonstrated a sudden onset and lasted for about 3 s, but were not accompanied by consciousness disturbance. The patient had about 15–20 attacks per day which became aggravated when she felt nervous or anxious. She also complained of uncoordinated gait and was susceptible to fall. She was diagnosed with epilepsy at a local hospital and irregularly took sodium valproate (500 mg twice daily). However, the symptoms did not relieve significantly. One year ago, she went to another clinic and the medicine was adjusted to magnesium valproate (500 mg twice daily) combined with levetiracetam (500 mg twice daily), and the limb tics relieved a little. Past medical history revealed that the patient presented multiple lipomas and pes cavus. Her older daughter (III₁) had a history of similar presentations and died at 16 years old (Fig. 2.5).

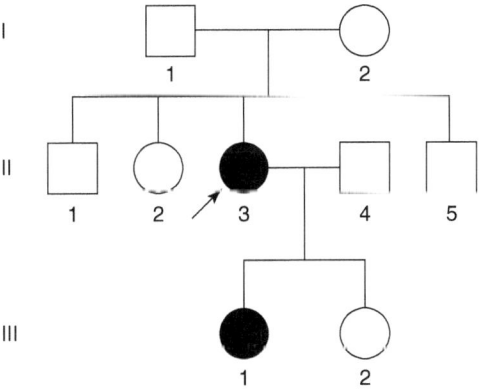

Fig. 2.5 Pedigree of the patient's family. *Squares* indicate males; *circles* indicate females; the *black symbols* indicate affected individuals; the *diagonal lines across symbol* indicate the deceased individual; the *arrow* indicates the proband

The neurological examinations showed a normal mental status and mild dysarthria. Examinations of the cranial nerves were unremarkable. Paroxysmal right upper limb tics were observed. Her muscle strength was graded 4–5 distally and 5 proximally. Muscular tone and sensory were normal. The patient with broad gait could not walk in a straight line. Romberg sign was positive. Babinski and Hoffman signs were absent.

The routine blood tests including white blood cell count, hematocrit, platelets, sodium, potassium, chloride, carbon dioxide, blood urea nitrogen, creatinine, glucose, and prothrombin time disclosed unremarkable findings. Immunology and rheumatism tests were negative. Electroencephalography (EEG) revealed spikes and slow waves.

Primary Diagnosis

A middle-aged woman was referred for problems with limb tics, weakness, and cerebellar ataxia, suggesting the impairment of cortex and cerebellum. The relatively long course of disease and positive family history implied the hereditary diseases should be considered first. Myoclonus was the most prominent feature of the patient over the entire course of the disease. The possible diagnosis consideration should include mitochondrial diseases, sialic acid storage disease, and neuronal ceroid lipofuscinoses (NCLs). Sialic acid storage disease is an autosomal recessive inherited disorder thus is excluded. Mitochondrial diseases involve multiple systems with variable clinical symptoms and recurrent episodes which cannot be excluded. NCLs are characterized with variable symptoms, including seizures, cerebral atrophy, dementia, and visual loss. Although most NCLs are autosomal recessive disorders, some autosomal dominant families were also reported. Additional tests including brain MRI, organic acid tests of the blood and urine, lactic acid test, and muscle biopsy were needed to further determine the diagnosis.

Additional Tests or Key Results

The brain MRI was normal. Basic lactic acid level from the blood was 4.4 mmol/L (reference

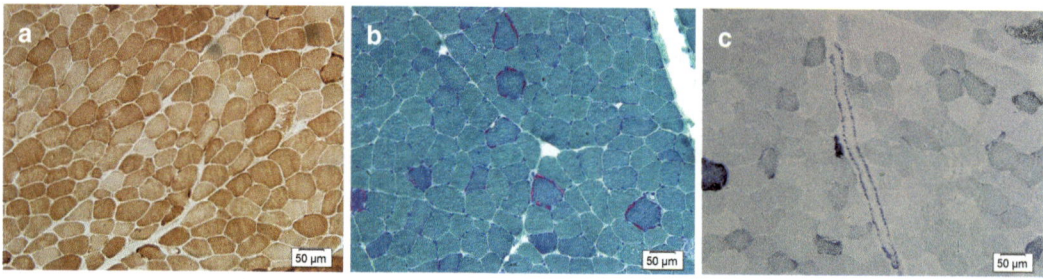

Fig. 2.6 Histologic staining of the muscle tissue from the patient shows several COX enzyme activity decreased or absent in muscle fibers using COX staining (**a**), positive MGT-staining RRFs (**b**), and strong SDH-reactive blood vessels (**c**) were found

Fig. 2.7 Chromatogram of m.8344A>G mutation detected in the patient

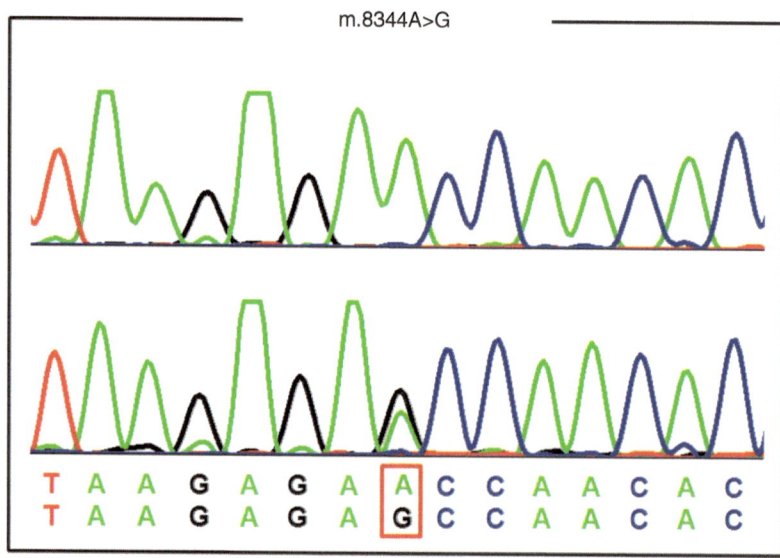

range 0.7–2.1 mmol/L), immediate blood lactic acid level after exercise was 6.8 mmol/L (reference range 0.7–2.1 mmol/L), and blood lactic acid level after 10 min rest was 5.3 mmol/L (reference range 0.7–2.1 mmol/L). Histologic staining of the muscle tissue from the patient shows several cytochrome c oxidase (COX) enzyme activities decreasing or absent in muscle fibers using COX staining (Fig. 2.6a). Ragged red fiber (RRF) was positive by modified Gomori trichrome (MGT) staining (Fig. 2.6b), and strong succinate dehydrogenase (SDH)-reactive blood vessels were found in the muscle tissue (Fig. 2.6c). The elevated lactic acid level and RRF found in muscle biopsy highly implied that the probable diagnosis was myoclonic epilepsy associated with ragged red fibers (MERRF).

Then we examined the most common mutation of MERRF. The sequencing of mtDNA was positive for m.8344A>G mutation thereby confirming the diagnosis of MERRF (Fig. 2.7).

Discussion

Mitochondrial diseases have versatile clinical and genetic aspects [5]. However, some specific syndromes are well understood like MERRF, which is a maternally inherited progressive multisystem syndrome usually beginning in childhood, but onset may also occur in adulthood. Patients with MERRF have several typical manifestations including myoclonus, generalized epilepsy, cerebellar ataxia, and RRF on muscle biopsy [6]. MERRF is caused by the mutations in mtDNA. The pathogenesis of the disease depends upon the proportion of mtDNA mutation, and the thresholds for dysfunction are different in various tissues. This is one of the reasons why mitochondrial diseases have versatile clinical manifestations. The myoclonus can occur independently or in association with generalized seizures in MERRF patient. MERRF predominantly affects gray matter, red nucleus, the inferior olivary nucleus, cerebellar dentate nucleus, and pons of the brainstem.

Here we demonstrated a typical case of MERRF with classical phenotype and genotype. The patient was misdiagnosed with epilepsy and treated with sodium valproate to control seizures for a long time. Sodium valproate is potentially mitochondrial poison which will increase the morbidity and mortality in patients with mitochondrial disease [7]. It is of particular importance to identify mitochondrial disease from other disease that can cause seizure. Similar with the patients with mitochondrial myopathy, encephalopathy, lactic acidosis, and a stroke-like episode (MELAS), the lactic acid level in the MERRF patient's blood and CSF is usually elevated at rest and can increase moderately after physical activity, but compared with MELAS patients, these levels are relatively low.

The muscle biopsy is an important diagnostic tool for MERRF because RRF are found in more than 90% of patients. Muscle fibers with deficient activity of COX imply that respiratory chain complex IV is one of the complexes that are most frequently impaired in MERRF patients. Mutation analysis of mtDNA is also important for MERRF diagnosis, and the most common mutation in MERRF patients is m.8344A>G [8].

There is no cure or specific treatment for MERRF. Treatment is limited to symptomatic and supportive management. The myoclonus improved markedly in 75% of patients treated with levetiracetam. Co-enzyme Q10 and L-carnitine have been used to ameliorate symptoms. Supportive management also includes additional therapy for complications such as cardiac disease, deafness, and diabetes mellitus. Genetic counseling and the option of genetic testing should be offered to at-risk relatives.

2.3 Cherry-Red Spot Myoclonus

A 13-Year-Old Boy Underwent 6 Years of Hypopsia and 2 Years of Limb Tic

Clinical Presentations

A 13-year-old boy came to our Neurology Clinic, complaining about progressive hypopsia for 6 years and unstable gait for 2 years. He had an unremarkable delivery and normal development milestones. His binocular vision became decreased when he was 7 years old. With difficulty in walking upstairs, he had to wear myopic lens for his blurred vision. At the age of 11, he experienced twitch of his limbs. The episodes usually lasted 2–3 min each time with loss of consciousness. Carbamazepine at a dose of 100 mg thrice daily was prescribed for him, but the events still occurred 3–5 times every year. Four months later, he exhibited gait difficulty and fall down to the ground sometimes. He could not hand the chopsticks steadily when picking up food. There was no complains of vertigo, dysphagia, or hypoacusis. His intelligence was intact and recognition was not impaired. He did not have any history of toxic exposure. His parents were not consanguineous; neither of them suffered similar symptoms.

Cranial nerve examinations revealed blurred vision, horizontal nystagmus, and visual field defect. His left visual acuity was 0.5/1.0, and right visual acuity was 0.6/1.0. His motor and sensory examination was normal. However, deep tendon reflexes were hyperactive throughout, with +++ at the biceps, triceps, and knees. Both Hoffmann sign and Babinski sign were bilaterally positive. Romberg sign and straight test were positive.

The blood cell counting, hepatic function, and thyroid hormones revealed uninformative. Rheumatism and immunology test demonstrated negative results. Folic acid and vitamin B12 were within normal range. Electroencephalogram (EEG) revealed high amplitude of spike waves and spike wave complex in both cerebral hemispheres. The brain MRI disclosed unremarkable findings.

Primary Diagnosis

The young patient presented with progressive hypoplasia, limb tics, and unstable gait. Neurological examinations revealed impaired vision, hyperreflexia, and cerebral ataxia. The location diagnosis was retina or optic nerve, pyramidal tract, cerebellum, and cerebral cortex, respectively. Taken together, these disclosed the extensive involvement of the nervous system. The early onset and progressive course of the disease suggest that heredity, metabolism, and intoxication may be the etiology of his symptoms. No exposure of toxicant substance or heavy metal excluded the consideration of intoxication. Therefore, hereditary and metabolic disease was the first consideration. Ophthalmofundoscope and visual evoked potential (VEP) test were needed for his hypopsia. Organic acid test from the blood or urine was needed to verify some metabolic disorders. Electromyologram (EMG) was needed to clarify if the peripheral nerve or muscle was involved.

Additional Tests or Key Results

Funduscopic examination showed bilateral macular cherry-red spots and nerve atrophy (Fig. 2.8a, b). Perimetry of the patient demonstrated visual defect of oculus dexter and sinister (Fig. 2.8c, d). VEP revealed that eye waveform was not recorded. Tandem mass spectrum analysis disclosed unremarkable findings. All the organic acid was normal in his urine. EMG test was uninformative. The decreased visual acuity, myoclonus, and cherry-red spots suggested that cherry-red spot myoclonus syndrome should be firstly considered.

The sequencing of *NEU*1 gene was performed, revealing that the patient harbored compound heterozygous c.544A>G (p.S182G) and c.1021C>T (p.R341X) mutation (Fig. 2.9). The further sequencing revealed the patient's father carried c.544A>G mutation, while his mother carried c.1021C>T mutation.

Discussion

Cherry-red spot myoclonus syndrome, also termed sialidosis type 1, is an autosomal recessive lysosomal storage disorder due to the deficit

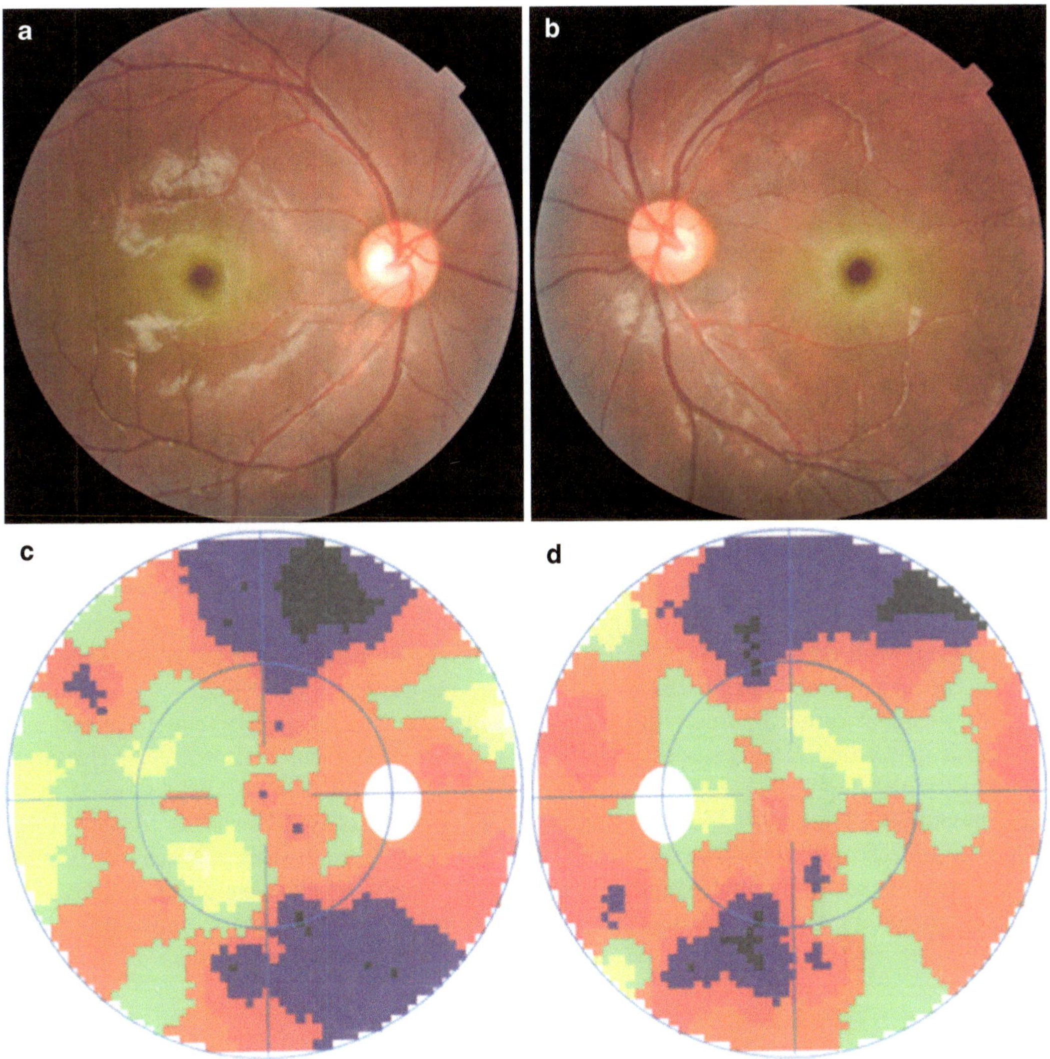

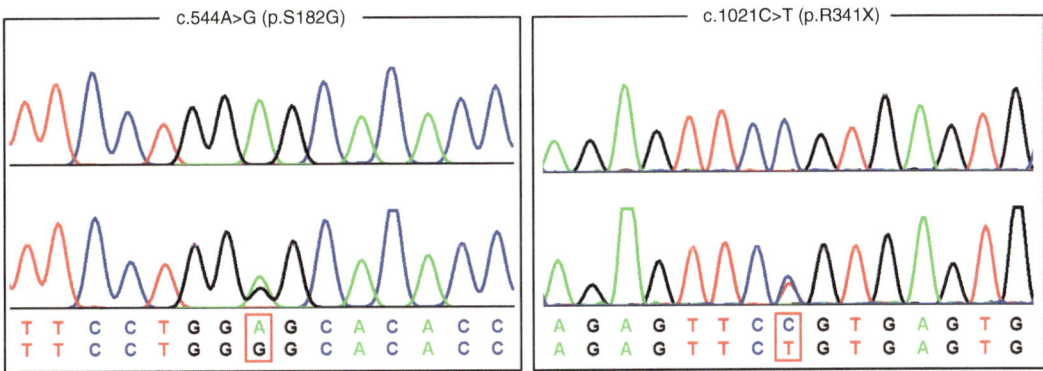

Fig. 2.8 Funduscopic examination revealed bilateral macular cherry-red spots and nerve atrophy (**a**, **b**). Perimetry of the patient demonstrated visual defect of oculus dexter (**c**) and sinister (**d**)

Fig. 2.9 Chromatogram of c.544A>G (p.S182G) (**a**) and c.1021C>T (p.R341X) (**b**) mutations within *NEU*1 gene. The *upper panel* indicates the normal sequence, the *lower panel* depicts mutated sequence

of neuraminidase [9]. It is an attenuated type of sialidosis and is characterized by myoclonus, visual impairment, and ataxia between the ages 20 and 30, without obvious physical or intelligence defects [10]. In contrast, sialidosis type II is a severe form of sialidosis, with infantile onset, coarse facial features, hepatomegaly, dysostosis multiplex, and mental retardation [11]. Although sialidosis type I and type II are both caused by *NEU*1 mutation, they are seemingly distinct diseases clinically. Sialidosis type II have an early onset, a rapid course, and a dismal prognosis, while type I present later in life with a mild disease that is mostly confined to vision, myoclonus, and minor neurologic manifestations.

The core symptoms in this case are hypopsia, myoclonus, and ataxia. Therefore, several diseases should be considered, including myoclonus epilepsy with ragged red fibers (MERRF), dentatorubral-pallidoluysian atrophy (DRPLA), Lafora, neuronal ceroid lipofuscinosis (NCL), sialidosis, and so on. The absence of exercise intolerance and intelligence deficit implied the less possibility of MERRF. DRPLA could be excluded because of the recessive inheritance in this family. The relatively mild symptoms without recognition impairment and slow course of disease were not consistent with the clinical

features of Lafora and NCL. The cherry-red spot sign is a crucial clue for the diagnosis in this case. However, this sign was not exclusive in sialidosis type I but was also described in GM1/GM2 gangliosidosis, Goldberg syndrome, Niemann-Pick disease, Wolman disease, and so on [12]. Combining cherry-red spot and myoclonus in this young girl, sialidosis type I should be considered. With the identification of *NEU*1 mutation in this case, the diagnosis of sialidosis type I could be made. If the ophthalmofundoscope was not performed or the funduscopic examination revealed unremarkable findings, the diagnosis in this case should include several other diseases.

Currently, there is no available therapy for sialidosis. Enzyme replacement therapy (ERT) is the classical therapeutic method for lysosomal storage disorders [13]. However, no ERT was successful in patients with sialidosis type I. A recombinant Neu1 enzyme was attempted in Neu1−/− mice, but elicited a severe immune response in the mutant mice [14, 15]. In addition, a pharmacologic chaperone-mediated therapy was successfully tested in the mouse model of type I sialidosis recently [16]. It was hypothesized that this approach may be effective for the *NEU*1 mutations found in patients with sialidosis type I. Levetiracetam is recommended to control the myoclonus in patients.

2.4 Tuberous Sclerosis Complex (TSC)

A 29-Year-Old Woman with Left Limb Numbness

Clinical Presentation

A 29-year-old woman presented with left limb numbness for over 10 days. She reported numbness descending from her left arm to her lower feet and could not walk steadily 5 days ago. She denied any eyelid drooping, blurred vision, chewing, or swallowing difficulty. She had a past medical history of moderate intellectual disability and seizures for over 10 years which was treated with antiepilepsy drug. Seizures were well controlled and did not recur in recent 5 years without antiepilepsy drug. There was no family history of note (Fig. 2.10).

Physical examination revealed multiple sebaceous adenomas appearing on her face and ungual fibroma appearing on her back (Fig. 2.11). The neurological examinations revealed a decreased cognitive abilities, which are evaluated by Mini-Mental State Examination (MMSE) and the score is 9/30. Examinations of the cranial nerves revealed unremarkable finding. Her

muscle strength was graded four on a scale of five distally of the left upper limb. Muscle tone was normal. She had a decreased sensation to pinprick and touch to left limbs. Tendon reflexes were normal. Babinski and Hoffman sign was negative. Her neck was supple and Kernig's sign was negative.

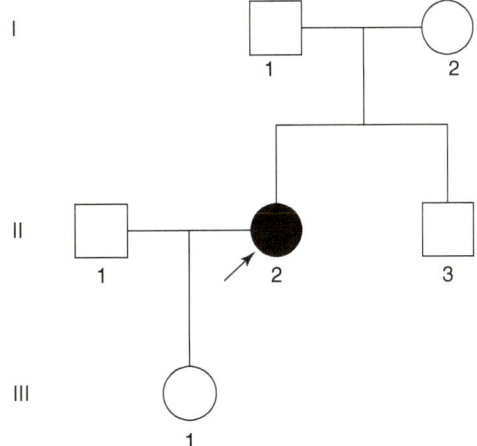

Fig. 2.10 The pedigree of the patient. *Squares* indicate males; *circles* indicate females; the *black symbols* indicate affected individuals; *diagonal lines across symbols* indicate deceased individuals; *arrows* indicate the probands

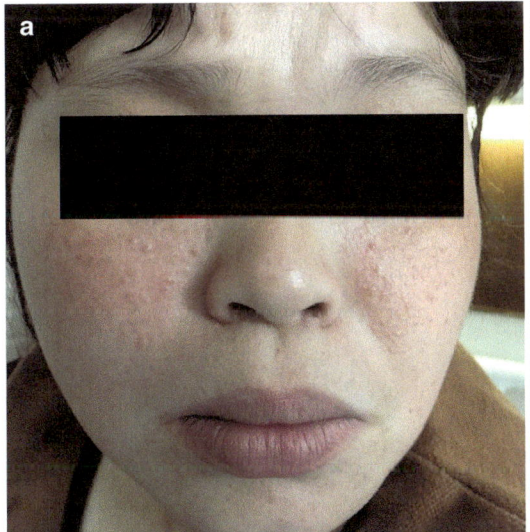
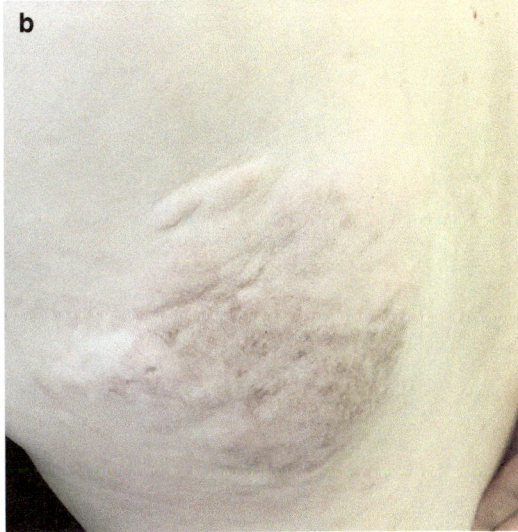

Fig. 2.11 Dermatologic manifestations of the patient. (**a**) Multiple sebaceous adenomas appearing on the patient's face and (**b**) ungual fibroma appearing on her back

The blood routine examination including white blood cell count, hematocrit, platelets, prothrombin time, blood urea nitrogen, creatinine, glucose, liver, and thyroid function disclosed unremarkable findings. Rheumatism and immunology test showed negative results. Erythrocyte sedimentation rate and C reactive protein were in the normal range.

Primary Diagnosis

The past medical history, symptoms, and signs of this patient hint the involvement of cognitive impairment, seizures, left limbs numbness, and mild muscle weakness as well as skin lesions which mean widespread cortex, suspected pyramidal tract, and the skin that was affected. Based on the long course of the disease, the neurologic symptoms, and skin lesions, neurocutaneous syndrome should be considered first for this patient. The differential diagnosis should include neurofibromatosis (NF), tuberous sclerosis complex (TSC), Sturge-Weber syndrome (SWS), and cerebral vascular disease. NF influences the growth and development of nerve cell tissue and is characterized by multiple cafe au lait spots and neurofibromas on the skin or in the brain. TSC is characterized by the presence of hamartomatous growths in multiple organs. The hallmark of SWS is a facial cutaneous venous dilation, typically in the distribution of the trigeminal nerve. Thus the brain CT should

be examined first. MRI scanning was necessary to exclude the cerebral vascular disease.

Additional Tests or Key Results

The brain CT revealed multiple intracranial high-density nodules (Fig. 2.12).

MRI scanning showed multiple nodules on both sides of the wall of the lateral ventricle with hypointense on both T1-weighted images and T2-weighted images (Fig. 2.13).

According to the neuroimaging results, combined with dermatologic manifestations, TSC should be considered first. Genetic testing was performed to detect the most common TSC-causative gene *TSC1*. The sequencing of *TSC1* revealed that the patient harbored *TSC1* c.1553delAGinsGAACT (p.K518Rfs*15) mutation thereby confirming the diagnosis of TSC (Fig. 2.14).

Discussion

TSC, also known as Bourneville disease, is a rare autosomal dominant neurocutaneous syndrome characterized by the presence of hamartomatous growths in multiple organs [17]. Hamartomas are frequently present in the brain, skin, kidneys, heart, and lung. Typical central nervous system (CNS) involvement includes subependymal nodules, cortical tubers, and benign white matter

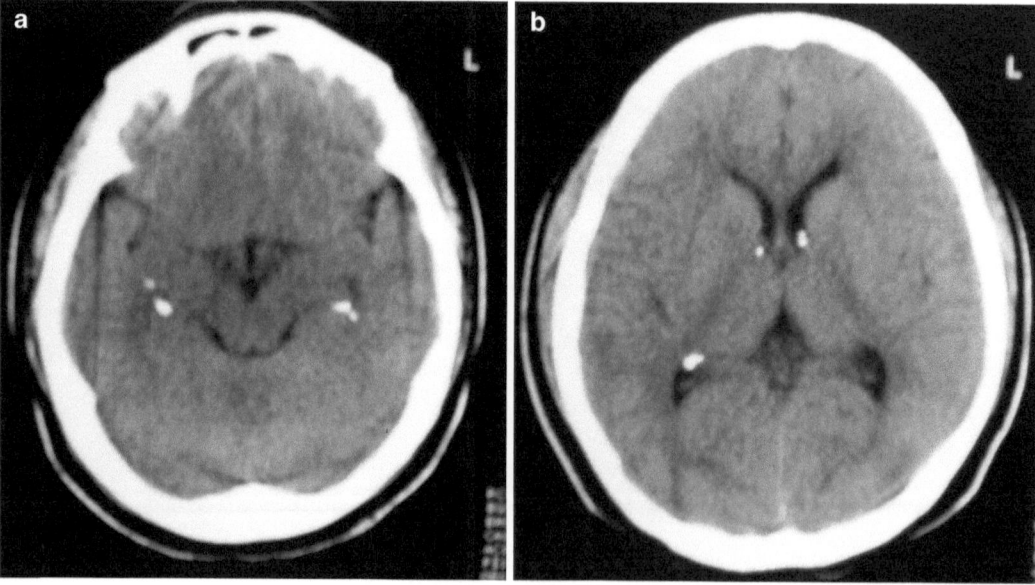

Fig. 2.12 Brain CT of the patient. Brain CT examination (**a**, **b**) showed multiple intracranial high-density nodules

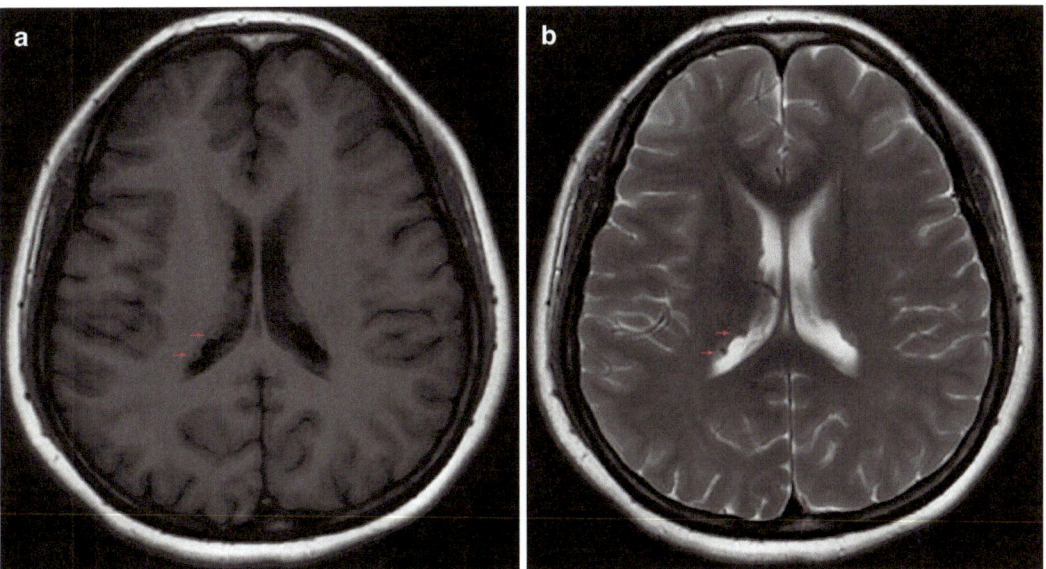

Fig. 2.13 Brain MRI of the patient. MRI examination showed multiple nodules on both sides of the wall of the lateral ventricle with hypointense on both T1-weighted (**a**) and T2-weighted images (**b**)

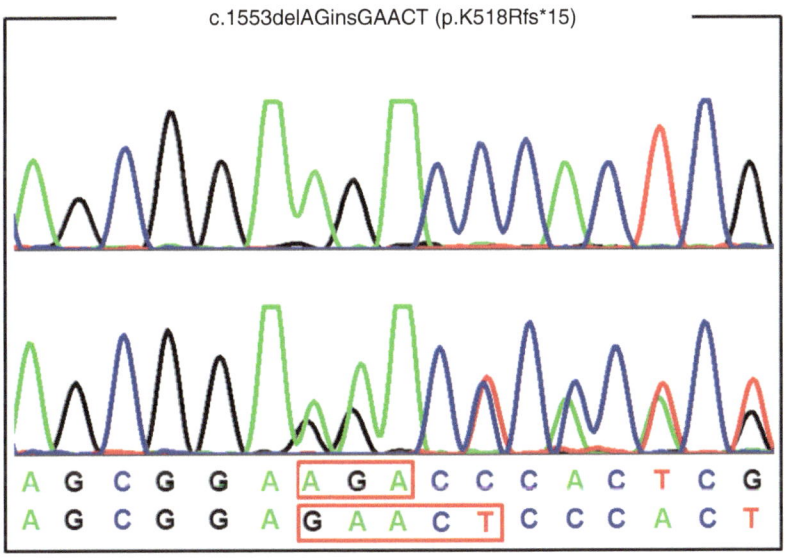

Fig. 2.14 Mutation analysis of the patient. The sequencing of TSC1 was positive for c.1553delAGinsGAACT (p.K518Rfs*15)

lesions. Tubers are composed of dysmorphic neurons occupying a cortical or subcortical location, showing abnormal signal on CT or MRI. Cortical tubers may calcify and approximately 50% of patients have calcified cortical tubers by age 10. Most TSC patients suffer from epilepsy and cognitive and behavioral problems.

In this case, the patient showed a typical clinical phenotype of TSC with cognitive impairment, seizures, and skin lesions. TSC most often presents with neurologic symptoms, with up to 90% of affected individuals experiencing seizures [18] and near half of the patients experiencing cognitive impairment [19]. Subependymal nodules are

found in nearly 95% of patients. Renal and dermatologic manifestations are also the common findings associated with TSC. In this case, kidney and
eye examination disclosed no positive finding.

TSC is caused by the mutation in either of the
two genes *TSC*1 and *TSC*2. A causative mutation
in *TSC*1 or *TSC*2 is identified in about 85% of
TSC patients [20]. Over 60% of cases are sporadic
and are considered to represent new mutations
[21]. *TSC*1 encodes hamartin, which forms an
intracellular complex inhibiting the target of
rapamycin (mTOR). mTOR is an ubiquitously
expressed protein that modulates cell proliferation
and growth, protein synthesis, and autophagy and
plays as a pivotal regulator of neuronal excitability. Genetic defect results in mTOR overactivation
which affects the normal cell growth and proliferation, neuronal excitability, and synaptogenesis
leading to epilepsy and neuropsychiatric disorders. *TSC*2 encodes a protein called tuberin which
has a GAP domain near the carboxy-terminal.
*TSC*1 and *TSC*2 interact physically to form het-
erodimers [22]. However, the clinical relevance of
these interactions is not yet well understood.

Currently there has been no specific therapy
for TSC. Symptomatic and supportive cares
including antiepilepsy, reducing intracranial
pressure, and facial angiofibroma treatment are
the mainstay treatment for patients. In animal
experiments, inhibitors of mTOR treated in the
early postnatal period before the first seizure
have a notable efficacy in preventing epilepsy
onset in rodents, but have no effect on long-term
sequelae including cognitive impairment and
development delay [23, 24]. Genetic counseling
and the option of genetic testing should be offered
to at-risk relatives.

References

1. Kraemer M, Berlit P. Primary central nervous system
   vasculitis and moyamoya disease: similarities and dif-
   ferences. J Neurol. 2010;257(5):816–819.
2. Mancuso M, Orsucci D, Angelini C, Bertini E, Carelli
   V, Comi GP, Donati A, Minetti C, Moggio M, Mongini
   T, Servidei S, Tonin P, Toscano A, Uziel G, Bruno C,
   Ienco EC, Filosto M, Lamperti C, Catteruccia M,
   Moroni I, Musumeci O, Pegoraro E, Ronchi D,
   Santorelli FM, Sauchelli D, Scarpelli M, Sciacco M,
   Valentino ML, Vercelli L, Zeviani M, Siciliano G. The
   m.3243A>G mitochondrial DNA mutation and
   related phenotypes. A matter of gender? J Neurol.
   2014;261(3):504–510.
3. El-Hattab AW, Adesina AM, Jones J, Scaglia F.
   MELAS syndrome: clinical manifestations, pathogenesis, and treatment options. Mol Genet Metab.
   2015;116(1–2):4–12.
4. Santa KM. Treatment options for mitochondrial
   myopathy, encephalopathy, lactic acidosis, and stroke-
   like episodes (MELAS) syndrome. Pharmacotherapy.
   2010;30(11):1179–1196.
5. Magner M, Kolarova H, Honzik T, Svandova I, Zeman
   J. Clinical manifestation of mitochondrial diseases.
   Dev Period Med. 2015;19(4):441–449.
6. DiMauro S, Hirano M. Merrf[A]. In: Pagon RA,
   Adam MP, Ardinger HH, Wallace SE, Amemiya A,
   Bean LJH, Bird TD, Ledbetter N, Mefford HC, Smith
   RJH, Stephens K, editors. GeneReviews(R). Seattle,
   WA: University of Washington; 1993.
7. Finsterer J, Zarrouk Mahjoub S. Mitochondrial toxicity of antiepileptic drugs and their tolerability in mitochondrial disorders. Expert Opin Drug Metab Toxicol.
   2012;8(1):71–79.
8. Lamperti C, Zeviani M. Myoclonus epilepsy in mitochondrial disorders. Epileptic Disord. 2016;18(S2):
   94–102.
9. Till JS, Roach ES, Burton BK. Sialidosis (neuraminidase deficiency) types I and II: neuro-ophthalmic
   manifestations. J Clin Neuroophthalmol. 1987;7(1):
   40–44.
10. Franceschetti S, Canafoglia L. Sialidosis. Epileptic
    Disord. 2016;18(S2):89–93.
11. Caciotti A, Di Rocco M, Filocamo M, Grossi S,
    Traverso F, d'Azzo A, et al. Type II sialidosis: review
    of the clinical spectrum and identification of a new
    splicing defect with chitotriosidase assessment in two
    patients. J Neurol. 2009;256(11):1911–1915.
12. Leavitt JA, Kotagal S. The "cherry red" spot. Pediatr
    Neurol. 2007;37(1):74–75.
13. d'Azzo A, Machado E, Annunziata I. Pathogenesis,
    emerging therapeutic targets and treatment in siali-
    dosis. Expert Opin Orphan Drugs. 2015;3(5):
    491–504.
14. Wang D, Bonten EJ, Yogalingam G, Mann L, d'Azzo
    A. Short-term, high dose enzyme replacement therapy
    in sialidosis mice. Mol Genet Metab. 2005;85(3):
    181–189.
15. Bonten EJ, Wang D, Toy JN, Mann L, Mignardot A,
    Yogalingam G, et al. Targeting macrophages with
    baculovirus-produced lysosomal enzymes: implica-
    tions for enzyme replacement therapy of the glyco-
    protein storage disorder galactosialidosis. FASEB
    J. 2004;18(9):971–973.
16. Bonten EJ, Yogalingam G, Hu H, Gomero E, van de
    Vlekkert D, d'Azzo A. Chaperone-mediated gene
    therapy with recombinant AAV-PPCA in a new mouse
    model of type I sialidosis. Biochim Biophys Acta.
    2013;1832(10):1784–1792.

17. Curatolo P, Moavero R, Roberto D, Graziola F. Genotype/phenotype correlations in tuberous sclerosis complex. Semin Pediatr Neurol. 2015;22(4):259–273.
18. Zaroff CM, Devinsky O, Miles D, Barr WB. Cognitive and behavioral correlates of tuberous sclerosis complex. J Child Neurol. 2004;19(11):847–852.
19. Thiele EA. Managing and understanding epilepsy in tuberous sclerosis complex. Epilepsia. 2010; 51(Suppl 1):90–1.
20. DiMario Jr FJ, Sahin M, Ebrahimi-Fakhari D. Tuberous sclerosis complex. Pediatr Clin N Am. 2015;62(3):633–648.
21. Jones AC, Shyamsundar MM, Thomas MW, Maynard J, Idziaszczyk S, Tomkins S, Sampson JR, Cheadle JP. Comprehensive mutation analysis of TSC1 and TSC2-and phenotypic correlations in 150 families with tuberous sclerosis. Am J Hum Genet. 1999;64(5):1305–1315.
22. Haddad LA, Smith N, Bowser M, Niida Y, Murthy V, Gonzalez-Agosti C, Ramesh V. The TSC1 tumor suppressor hamartin interacts with neurofilament-L and possibly functions as a novel integrator of the neuronal cytoskeleton. J Biol Chem. 2002;277(46):44180–186.
23. Costa V, Aigner S, Vukcevic M, Sauter E, Behr K, Ebeling M, Dunkley T, Friedlein A, Zoffmann S, Meyer CA, Knoflach F, Lugert S, Patsch C, Fjeldskaar F, Chicha-Gaudimier L, Kiialainen A, Piraino P, Bedoucha M, Graf M, Jessberger S, Ghosh A, Bischofberger J, Jagasia R. mTORC1 inhibition corrects neurodevelopmental and synaptic alterations in a human stem cell model of tuberous sclerosis. Cell Rep. 2016;15(1):86–95.
24. Way SW, Rozas NS, Wu HC, McKenna 3rd J, Reith RM, Hashmi SS, Dash PK, Gambello MJ. The differential effects of prenatal and/or postnatal rapamycin on neurodevelopmental defects and cognition in a neuroglial mouse model of tuberous sclerosis complex. Hum Mol Genet. 2012;21(14): 3226–3236.

Li-Xi Li, Zhi-Jun Liu, Wan-Jin Chen,
Hong-Xia Wang, Hong-Lei Li, and Sheng Chen

Abstract

Motor neuron disease (MND) is a group of neurological disorders which is characterized by selectively progressive degeneration of motor neurons in the brain and spinal cord. On the basis of the degree of upper or lower neuron involvement, MND is broadly divided into several subtypes: pure upper neuron diseases (primary lateral sclerosis), pure lower motor neuron diseases (progressive spinal muscular atrophy, progressive bulbar palsy, spinal muscular atrophy, X-linked spinal and bulbar muscular atrophy, etc.), and mixed upper and lower motor neuron diseases (amyotrophic lateral sclerosis). Generally, MND can be sporadic, or it can occur as an inherited disorder. To date, a great number of genes have been identified to be responsible for inherited MND. The distinct causative genes usually result in different clinical phenotypes. Therefore, the genetic testing is crucial for inherited MND. In this chapter, we mentioned several cases of inherited motor neuron diseases and described the way how these definitive causative genes were identified. In addition, to make clear definition for MND, several other inherited neurologic diseases, such as hereditary spasticity paraplegia and inherited peripheral neuropathy, were also presented in this chapter.

Keywords

Motor neuron disease • Amyotrophic lateral sclerosis • Hereditary spastic paraplegia • Spinal muscular atrophy • Familial amyloidotic polyneuropathy • Charcot-Marie-Tooth disease • Kennedy's disease • Molecular diagnosis

L.-X. Li (✉) • Z.-J. Liu • H.-L. Li • S. Chen
Department of Neurology and Research Center of
Neurology, Second Affiliated Hospital, Zhejiang
University School of Medicine, Hangzhou, China
e-mail: llxidavy@hotmail.com

W.-J. Chen
Department of Neurology and Institute of Neurology,
First Affiliated Hospital, Fujian Medical University,
Fuzhou, China

H.-X. Wang
Department of Neurology, The First Affiliated
Hospital of Soochow University, Suzhou, China

© Springer Nature Singapore Pte Ltd. 2017
Z.-Y. Wu (ed.), *Inherited Neurological Disorders*, DOI 10.1007/978-981-10-4196-9_3

3.1 Amyotrophic Lateral Sclerosis (ALS)

A 49-Year-Old Male with Progressive Limbs Weakness and Muscle Atrophy

Clinical Presentations

A 49-year-old man came to our department with a history of over 20 years of progressive limbs weakness associated with muscle atrophy. He was first noted mild weakness of his bilateral legs at the age of 29. He gradually experienced difficulty in walking. Five years later, his arms were affected as well, with difficulty in lifting a heavy load over his head. In the next five years, he had increased difficulty in handgrip and walking. Obvious muscle atrophy was observed in both hands and legs. The disease affected his speech muscles when he was 43 years old. He exhibited a mild dysarthria but still had a relatively unimpaired swallowing ability. His cognition and behavior ability were not impaired during the entire disease course. The patient first started to take riluzole at the age of 49, though with a limit effect. More supportive care was currently home provided to enhance the quality of life.

Physical examinations on his first visit showed obvious atrophy of his bilateral intrinsic hand muscles and diffusely brisk deep tendon reflexes. Babinski sign was present bilaterally at the moment. In his recent examinations, positive signs included mild dysarthria, muscle weakness of both upper limbs and lower extremities. Muscle weakness involved all his extremities, with a decreased strength of the upper extremities (3–4/5) and lower extremities (2–4/5, distal weaken than proximal). The gag reflex was normal. Tendon reflexes were disappeared in all four extremities. Pathogenic signs weren't observed at this moment. His sensory and cerebellar function was normal. His cognition was evaluated normal as well.

The former medical history was unremarkable, apart from a record of slightly increased level of blood sugar. In total, six persons were affected by this disease in the family. They experienced the similar problems in their 20s (Fig. 3.1) and died of respiratory failure within a couple of years after onset. His younger sister developed limbs wasting at the age of 32 and underwent dysarthria at age 45.

There are no specific clinical findings on routine laboratory examinations. The blood tests showed unremarkable findings. Serum levels of T3, T4, and TSH were in normal range. Both folic acid and vitamin B12 were within normal range. There were no significant findings on test for rheumatoid factor and assessment of immunology system. The brain and cervical spinal magnetic resonance imaging (MRI) examination revealed unspecific findings. There were no abnormal findings on electroencephalography. Electromyography test showed extensive denervation in limb muscles and thoracic paraspinal muscles.

Primary Diagnosis

In this case, the patient mainly presented with slow progressive limbs weakness and severe

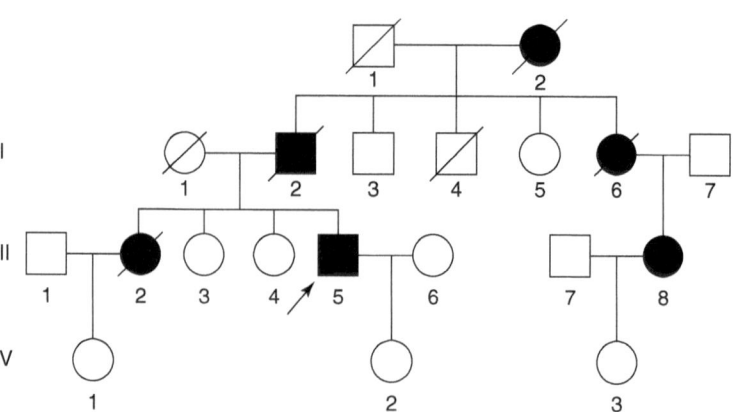

Fig. 3.1 The family pedigree of the patient. The *black field* indicates affected individuals; *circle*, female; *square*, male; *diagonal line* across symbol, deceased; *arrow*, proband

muscle atrophy, which were evidences of lower motor neuron deficits. EMG results also highly suggested the involvement of lower motor neuron. The Babinski signs observed in early stage indicated the entanglement of the upper motor neuron. Taken together, the clinical picture hinted the impairment of upper and lower motor neuron. Owing to the feature of midlife-onset and slowly progressive course in this patient, the diagnosis consideration should include the disturbance of neoplasm, metabolism, chronic inflammation, degeneration, and hereditary. Neoplasm could be excluded on the basis of the unspecific MRI findings and blood tests. Normal laboratory testing results basically ruled out the possibility of metabolism and chronic inflammation. Both upper and lower motor neuron were affected in the present case, indicated the deficits of the motor neuron processes. Therefore, the diagnosis of probable amyotrophic lateral sclerosis (ALS) could be made on the basis of revised El Escorial criteria [1]. The differential diagnosis also included lesions of cervical spine, multifocal motor neuropathy (MMN), and other forms of motor neuron diseases. Unremarkable MRI examination in the brain and spinal cord basically excluded the possibility of structural lesions of these sites. Multifocal motor neuropathy had typical electrophysiologic features of conduction block, which could be detected by nerve conduction examination. The multiple neurological examinations could provide more strong evidence of UMN impairment and help distinguish MND from other LMN disorders. Moreover, a positive family history was obviously observed in the disease with an autosomal-dominant pattern. Therefore, the genetic testing was required to unearth the genetic cause and help make the correct diagnosis.

Additional Tests or Key Results

Through targeted sequencing by combining the genes responsible for ALS in a custom panel, the patient was detected with a novel c.175G>C (p. G59R) mutation in *DCTN1* gene. The novel mutation was further certificated through Sanger sequencing in his affected younger sister (Fig. 3.2).

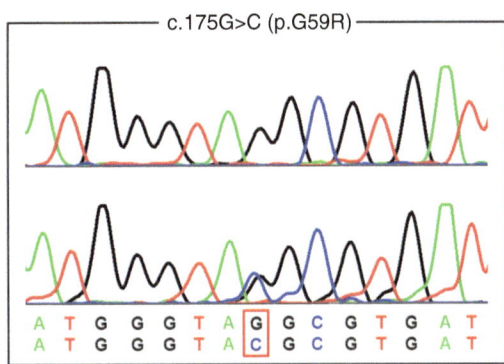

Fig. 3.2 Mutation analysis of the patient. Chromatogram of c.175G>C (p.G59R) mutation in *DCTN1*. The upper panel indicates the normal *DCTN1* sequence, whereas the lower panel shows the heterozygous mutated sequence

Discussion

ALS is manifested by progressive degeneration of both upper and lower motor neurons located in the cerebral cortex, brainstem, and spinal cord. This disease is first described by Jean-Martin Charcot in 1874 and become well recognized because of the two famous persons with ALS, Lou Gehrig and Stephen William Hawking, and increasingly common today due to the prevalence of ice bucket challenge in 2012. The typical symptoms comprise muscle weakness, muscular atrophy, pyramidal tract signs, and the absence of sensory impairment. The average age onset of ALS is 65 years [2]. Most patients die from failure of respiration within 3–5 years after the onset, but about 10% of patients may still survive as much as 10 years and even longer. Unlike classical ALS, which tends to affect people with a rapidly progression, the clinical feature of the present patient was atypical. In this case, the course of the disease was slowly progressive, with a period of 13 years from limbs onset to bulbar symptom. In his family, his affected younger sister also experienced the similar slow course of progression. During the early stage of the disease, upper motor signs were identified in our case; nevertheless, lower motor signs were the primarily symptoms in the whole disease course. This suggests a wide variability of UMN and LMN involvement in the whole process of ALS. Given the critical role of involvement of both UMN and LMN in ALS diagnosis, careful neurological examinations should be performed at different stages of the disease.

About 5–10% of ALS patients show familial inherited pattern (autosomal-dominant or autosomal-recessive inheritance). More than 19 disease-causing genes have been described in familial ALS (FALS) [3]. Among them, *SOD1*, *TDP-43*, and *FUS* make up about 30% in all FALS cases [4]. Moreover, ALS is also a kind of disease with highly genetic heterogeneity and clinical variability. Different causative genes can still result in similar phenotypes in ALS patients. Therefore, it is a big challenge to identify underlying mutations with traditional sequencing method. Targeted sequencing, a new relatively rapid and economic molecular diagnosis strategy, makes it possible to screen culprit genes or mutations in FALS patients.

The patient was finally detected with *DCTN1* mutation through targeted sequencing. The first mutation of *DCTN1* related to MND was reported in 2003, and several *DCTN1* mutations were described in families affected with ALS or ALS-FTD. However, there was an obvious variability with regard to the associated phenotypes of *DCTN1* mutations. The severity of disease and the course of disease are varied largely among the interfamilial or intrafamilial members with *DCTN1* mutations.

The pathogenic mechanism of ALS is believed to be utmost complicate, which would involve multiple mechanisms. Although huge improvement has been made to elucidate the mechanisms of ALS during the past two decades, the specific mechanism is still unclear. To date, there is no effective medical treatment for ALS. Many drugs that have been initially developed and showed a promise in the field of cure ALS, but the majority of them failed the final clinical trial.

3.2   Hereditary Spastic Paraplegia (HSP)

A 24-Year-Old Male with 10-Years History of Abnormal Gait

Clinical Presentations

A 24-year-old man came to our neurological department with a chief complaint of abnormal gait for over 10 years. He had gait disturbance at the age of 14. The symptoms progressed slowly and became evident in the last 3 years. He felt weak in the lower limbs and had difficulty in going downstairs because of his stiff legs. The upper limbs were intact. He denied cognitive impairment, headaches, eyelid drooping, double vision, swallowing difficulty, or shortness of breath. He did not complain urinary bladder incontinence. He had no other medical problems and was not taking any medications. The patient was of Chinese descent, and his mother also developed gait disturbance at the age of 35 (Fig. 3.3a).

The neurological examination showed higher muscle tone, increased reflexes in the lower limbs, positive bilateral Babinski sign, and ankle clonus. His gait was stiff with scissoring. He had difficulties with tandem gait. His speech is fluent. No cognitive impairment, abnormal signs of cranial nerves, or extrapyramidal disturbances were observed. Strength and sensory examinations in upper extremities were normal. No muscle weakness, muscle atrophy, or sensory deficits in the lower limbs was noted. Romberg test and finger-to-nose test were negative. No scoliosis or kyphoscoliosis was observed.

The routine laboratorial screening tests, including routine blood test, blood biochemical test, vitamin B12, folate, C-reactive protein (CRP), erythrocyte sedimentation rate (ESR), and thyroid

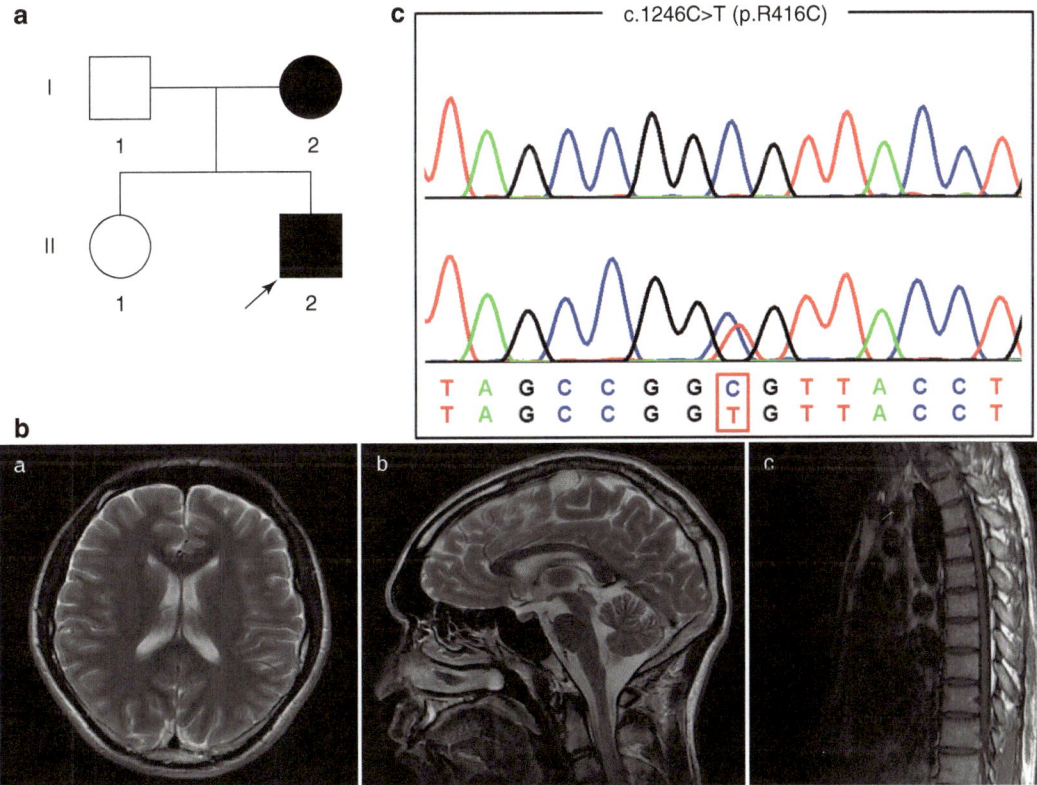

Fig. 3.3 The pedigree, MRI examination and sequencing chromatograms. (**a**) The pedigree of the patient. *Arrow* indicates the proband. The *black box* indicates the affected patient. (**b**) The brain and spinal cord MRI examination indicate normal structure. (**c**) The sequencing chromatograms reveal a heterozygous variant c.1246C>T of the *ATL1* gene in the patient

function, were within normal ranges. The examination of a group of autoantibodies, such as antinuclear antibodies, anti-double-stranded DNA antibodies, and anti-Smith antibodies, was negative. Serology for HIV, hepatitis, and syphilis were negative as well. The X-ray examination for knee joint and hip joint was normal. No abnormalities were found in brain magnetic resonance imaging (MRI) examination (Fig. 3.3b).

Primary Diagnosis

Lower extremity spasticity, high muscle tone, hyperreflexia, positive Babinski sign, and absence of sensory impairment suggested the pyramidal dysfunction. The normal brain MRI findings and intact function of upper limbs hinted the involvement of the spinal cord below the cervical enlargement. As the patient's mother also had symptom of gait disturbance indicating a clear family history, an inherited disease affecting the spinal cord should be verified. The following diseases should be taking into account: familial amyotrophic lateral sclerosis, primary lateral sclerosis, structural abnormalities of spinal cord, spinocerebellar ataxias (SCA), hereditary spastic paraplegias (HSP), inherited metabolic diseases (homocysteine remethylation defects, arginase deficiency, etc.), and subacute combined degeneration of spinal cord.

Additional Tests or Key Results

The examination of thoracic spinal cord MRI, CSF analysis, and electrophysiological study were further performed. No abnormalities were found in spinal cord MRI examination (Fig. 3.3b). The nerve conduction studies and electromyography assessments were normal as well. The lumbar puncture with cerebrospinal fluid (CSF) analysis showed normal protein, glucose, cell counts, and IgG synthesis rate.

Since the serum vitamin B12 level, CSF analysis, and MRI examination of the spinal cord were normal, the disease of myelopathy (metabolic, compression) and structural abnormalities disorders were unlikely. Owing to long-term disease course, normal neurological examination in the upper extremities, and normal neurophysiologic test, amyotrophic lateral sclerosis was excluded. For inborn disorders of metabolism, the inheritance pattern is often an autosomal-recessive trait, and the clinical picture is usually not restricted to pyramidal signs [5]. Moreover, the level of serum homocysteine was normal. Therefore, inherited metabolic diseases were not primarily under consideration. The negative result of ATXN3 analysis, the gene responsible for SCA3, helps us to exclude the disease of SCA3. As HSP is the most common disease responsible for hereditary lower limb spasticity [6], we pay our attention to this disease.

Genomic DNA of this patient was extracted from peripheral EDTA-treated blood. A gene panel covering the causative gene associated with HSP was designed (Table 3.1). Targeted next-generation sequencing was further performed. After filtering, a heterozygous variant in ATL1

Table 3.1 The genes responsible for HSP were included in the gene panel

Disease	Gene	Disease	Gene	Disease	Gene	Disease	Gene
SPG1	L1CAM	SPG18	ERLIN2	SPG45	NT5C2	SPG59	USPS
SPG2	PLP1	SPG20	SPG20	SPG46	GBA2	SPG60	WDR48
SPG3A	ATL1	SPG21	ACP33	SPG47	AP4B1	SPG61	ARL6IP1
SPG4	SPAST	SPG22	SLC16A2	SPG48	AP5Z1	SPG62	ERLIN1
SPG5A	CYP7B1	SPG26	B4GALNT1	SPG49	TECPR2	SPG63	AMPD2
SPG6	NIPA1	SPG28	DDHD1	SPG50	AP4M1	SPG64	ENTPD1
SPG7	PGN	SPG30	KIF1A	SPG51	AP4E1	SPG65	NT5C2
SPG8	KIAA0196	SPG31	REEP1	SPG52	AP4S1	SPG66	ARS
SPG10	KIF5A	SPG33	ZFYVE27	SPG53	VPS37A	SPG67	PGAP1
SPG11	SPG11	SPG35	FA2H	SPG54	DDHD2	SPG68	FLRT1
SPG12	RTN2	SPG39	PNPLA6	SPG55	C12orf65	SPG69	RAB3GAP2
SPG13	HSPD1	SPG42	SLC33A1	SPG56	CYP2U1	SPG70	MARS
SPG15	ZFYVE26	SPG43	C19orf12	SPG57	TFG	SPG71	ZFR
SPG17	BSCL2	SPG44	GJC2	SPG58	KIF1C	SPG72	REEP2

c.1246C>T was identified which was confirmed by Sanger sequencing (Fig. 3.3c). This variant had been reported previously as pathogenic in HSP families [7]. Further sequencing demonstrated that the proband's mother had the same heterozygous variant in *ATL1*. Therefore, the patient was diagnosed with HSP.

Discussion

Hereditary spastic paraplegias (HSP), also termed spastic paraplegias (SPG), is a genetically and clinically heterogeneous group of neurological disorders which is commonly characteristic with progressive spasticity, extremities weakness, and some dorsal column impairment [8]. Postmortem studies of HSP patients indicated a length-dependent degeneration of the longest axons in the corticospinal tract [9]. HSP is clinically divided into two forms, pure HSP and complex HSP. Besides the corticospinal signs, other neurological signs may present in complicated HSP, such as ataxia, cognitive impairment, epilepsy, peripheral neuropathy, thin corpus callosum, and optic atrophy.

Up to now, at least 55 causative genes have been found to be associated with HSP [6, 8]. The transmission modes of HSP include autosomal-dominant (AD), autosomal-recessive (AR), X-linked, and maternal trait of inheritance [10]. Due to the genetic heterogeneity of HSP, it is difficult for the neurologist to detect all of the candidate genes to make a molecular diagnosis. Targeted next-generation sequencing, a high-throughput DNA sequencing technology that performs parallel sequencing of the genomic regions of interest, makes it possible to sequence thousands of genes [11]. Using this technology, we quickly detected the causative gene in this family.

Spastic paraplegia 3 (SPG3) is one of the most frequent autosomal-dominant type of HSP and is related to *ATL1* gene on chromosome 14q12-q2 [12]. The age of onset of SPG3 is around 4 years old and is rarely later than that age [13, 14]. Most SPG3 patients have a pure HSP phenotype [15]. Our patient also displayed a pure form HSP but with a late age of onset. The signs of vibration sensation deficits at the ankles and urinary sphincter hyperactivity were less frequently happened in SPG3. Accordingly, our patient did not show these two symptoms.

Treatment for HSP is exclusively symptomatic. Fortunately, the progression of HSP is slow, and wheelchair dependency is relatively rare. The goal of symptomatic treatment is to improve mobility and relieve the discomfort associated with spasticity. Medical therapy of spasticity may begin with oral baclofen. When the oral drugs are useless, intramuscular injections of botulinum toxin can be further under consideration. Moreover, the physical therapy concentrated on strengthening exercises should be combined with the pharmacotherapy [16, 17]. Genetic counseling for patients and their family is considerable.

3.3 Spinal Muscular Atrophy (SMA)

A 31-Year-Old Male with Progressive Muscle Weakness and Atrophy

Clinical Presentations

A 31-year-old man admitted to our hospital presented with progressive lower and upper limbs' muscular weakness for 20 years and aggravated these 5 years. He noted lower limbs' muscle weakness 20 years ago, manifested with difficulty in raising the stairs and running. This manifestation was progressive gradually, and the upper limbs also involved. During the last 5 years, these manifestations significantly aggravated, and now he is having difficulty in walking and cannot raise his arms, complicated with muscle atrophy in his upper and lower limbs. Medical history was unremarkable.

Neurological examinations revealed that cranial nerves were negative, without tongue muscle atrophy and fasciculation. Muscle atrophy was observed in his proximal limbs. Manual muscle testing (MMT, 0–5 grade) showed weakness of neck muscle (5- grade), upper proximal muscles (4 grade), and lower proximal muscles (2 grade), and the distal limb muscle strength was 5 grade. His muscular tension was decreased. All his upper and lower limbs' deep tendon reflexes were disappeared. Hoffmann, Babinski, and Romberg signs were bilaterally negative. His deep and superficial sensation examinations were symmetric and normal.

The blood routine examination was normal. Aspartate amino transferase (AST) was 55 U/L (normal range 0–50 U/L). Serum creatine kinase (CK) was 1435 U/L (normal range 55–170), and isoenzymes of creatine kinase (CK-MB) was 78 U/L (normal range <25 U/L). Serum lactate dehydrogenase (LDH) was 823 U/L (normal range 313–618 U/L). ECG test was normal without arrhythmia. Lung function test showed that FVC was 91.8%. The brain MRI disclosed unremarkable findings.

Interestingly, one of his uncles also presented with similar manifestations (Fig. 3.4a). He was 59 years old and noted lower limbs' muscle weakness at his age of 4. The muscle weakness progressed gradually as well as the upper limbs. At age of 30, he was unable to walk without assistant and needed crutch when walking. He was wheelchair dependent when he was 50 years old. Neurological examinations showed cranial nerves were negative. Muscle atrophy was observed, especially in his proximal limbs. MMT showed weakness of neck muscle (4 grade), upper proximal muscles (0–1 grade), upper distal muscles (3 grade), and lower limbs' muscles (0 grade). His muscular tension was decreased. All limbs' deep tendon reflexes were disappeared. Hoffmann and Babinski signs, as well as sensation examinations, were normal.

Primary Diagnosis

The patient showed muscle weakness and atrophy at all of the limbs, especially the proximal muscles. The muscle tension and deep tendon reflexes were disappeared, without Hoffmann and Babinski signs. The CK level was mildly increased. These symptoms, signs, and investigations hint the impairment of peripheral nervous system, and the localization of lesion should be considered from muscle, neuromuscular joint, to lower motor neurons.

The muscle weakness and atrophy was childhood onset, with a progressive course and positive family history, all of which implied that hereditary neurological diseases should be considered first for this patient, such as progressive muscular dystrophy (PMD), spinal muscular atrophy (SMA), and Kenney's disease (KD).

Additional Tests or Key Results

Electromyography (EMG) test revealed extensive neurogenic lesions, without conduction block. After informed consent, the proband also performed a muscle biopsy, the result of which further confirmed the neurogenic lesions (Fig. 3.4b). The childhood-onset progressive muscular weakness and atrophy, decrease muscle tension, and deep tendon reflexes, combined with neurogenic lesions from EMG and histopathological tests, strongly suggested the diagnosis of SMA. Thus, genetic test of survival of motor neuron 1 gene (*SMN1*) was carried out by poly-

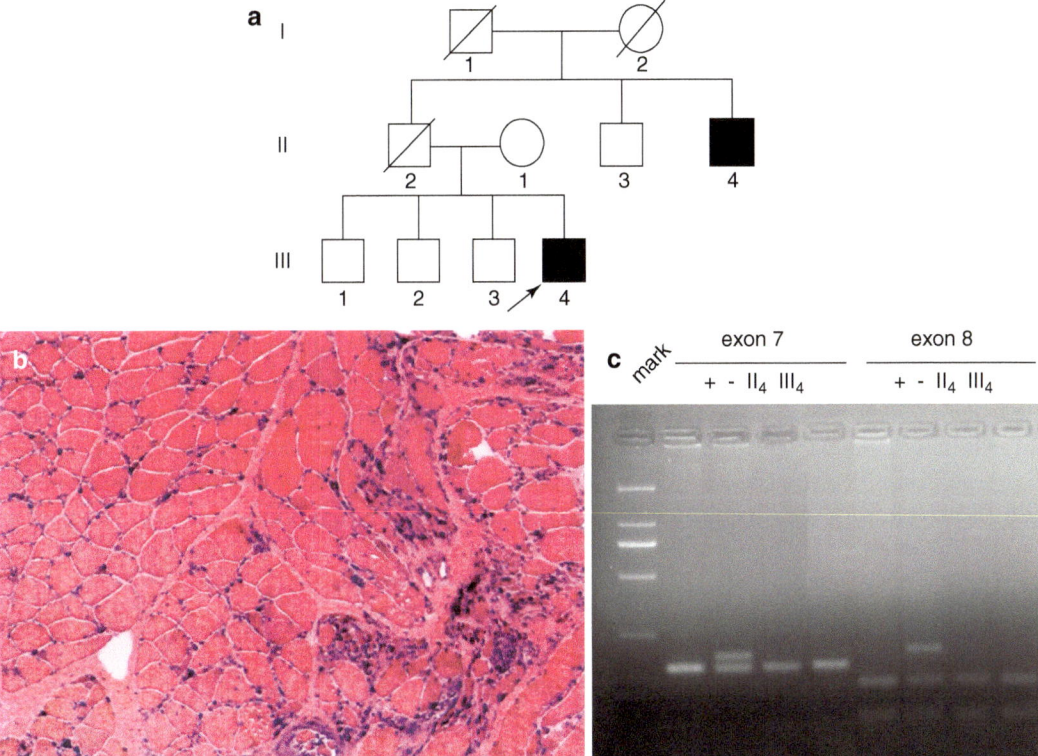

Fig. 3.4 (**a**) The patient's pedigree chart. *Arrow* indicates the proband; *square*, males; *circle*, females; *filled symbol*, affected individual; *diagonal lines* across symbol, deceased individual. (**b**) Muscle biopsy pathological examination showed neurogenic lesions by HE staining.

(**c**) Detection of *SMN1* and *SMN2* genes by PCR-RFLP. Both the proband (III_4) and his uncle (II_4) possessed the homozygous deletion of exons 7 and 8 in *SMN1* gene. *Plus*, positive control. *Minus*, negative control

merase chain reaction-restriction fragment length polymorphism (PCR-RFLP). Both the proband and his affected uncle carried the similar homozygous deletion of exon 7 and exon 8 (Fig. 3.4c).

Discussion

Childhood-onset SMA is an autosomal-recessive neurological disorder in humans with a high frequency of 1.4/10,000 and a carrier frequency of 1/42 in the mainland of China [18]. It is featured by selective degeneration of motor neurons in the spinal cord and progressive muscular weakness and atrophy. Based on onset age and motor function achieved, childhood-onset SMA can be classified into three types, SMA I–III [19]. Patients with SMA I, the most severe type, usually develop muscular weakness before 6 months and die within the first 2 years because of respiratory

failure. Patients with SMA II, the intermediate type, usually show onset after 6 months. Patients can sit but not walk without help, and their life span is significantly reduced. Patients with SMA III, the mild type, show onset after 18 months. They are able to walk but not run, and they become wheelchair bound during adulthood.

The causative gene, *SMN1*, was identified in 1995 [20]. Interestingly, survival of motor neuron 2 gene (*SMN2*), a highly identical homolog to *SMN1* in 5q13, modifies the disease severity and represents a promising therapeutic target for SMA now. *SMN1* and *SMN2* are highly identical, and the main difference is a C to T substitution at the 840 position of exon 7, which alters a Dra I enzyme site. Besides, a G to A substitution at the 236 position of exon 8 also creates a Dde I enzyme site. The Dra I and Dde I enzyme sites could be used to distinguish *SMN1* and *SMN2* by PCR-RFLP technology.

In this SMA family, the proband and his affected uncle showed their first symptoms at the age of 10 and 4, respectively, indicating that they were type III SMA patients. Besides, both of them showed typically clinical features for SMA, including progressive muscle weakness and atrophy, especially the proximal limbs, disappeared deep tendon reflexes, neurogenic lesions in EMG, and histopathological tests, as well as the deletion of *SMN1* gene. However, they possessed a similar disease course. Previously, we reported two rare families with two SMA patients in two continuous generations, but their symptoms were significantly different, which correlated with the copy number of *SMN2* gene [21]. In conclusion, this is a typical SMA pedigree, and we hope it will facilitate the understanding and diagnosis of SMA for clinical neurologists.

To date, no effective treatment is available for SMA. Recently, a set of drugs rendering the inclusion of exon 7 in *SMN2* gene were under investigated, including histone deacetylase inhibitors (HDACi), hydroxyurea, ceftriaxone, antisense oligo, and new synthetic compounds [22–24]. Weihl et al. [25] reported seven type III/IV SMA patients who were treated with valproate (VPA) and showed an increase of muscle strength and subjective function. However, in the following several large clinical trials, VPA or VPA plus L-carnitine failed to improve muscle strength or motor abilities in SMA patients [26–29]. The induced pluripotent stem (iPS) cell technology and CRISPR/Cas9 technology may be the new treatments for SMA in the future to achieve the cell replacement and gene correction [30–32].

3.4 Familial Amyloidotic Polyneuropathy (FAP)

A 45-Year-Old Female with Progressive Paresthesia and Limb Muscle Atrophy

Clinical Presentations

The patient was a 45-year-old woman who had progressive paresthesia for 4 years and weakness for 2 years in her four limbs. She developed stabbing, burning pain, and numbness at her pelma at age 41. The symptoms progressed slowly and extended up to knees in the next two years. Weakness and atrophy in her bilateral lower extremities and numbness in two hands were found afterward. She needed aid to walk and suffered from orthostatic hypotension, dry skin, and skin ulcer when she was transferred to our clinic at age 45. On further questioning, she reported visual problem since the age of 43. She

was diagnosed with peripheral neuropathy in local hospital. Methycobal and idebenone were administrated in the course of disease, but no effect was found in stopping the progression of the disease. Her condition continually worsened. Her developmental milestone was unremarkable. The patient had no past history of chronic diseases, such as diabetes and hypertension. She had no history of neurotoxin exposure. The patient's nephew, sister, father, uncles, aunts, and grandfather had similar symptoms (Fig. 3.5).

Physical examinations showed orthostatic hypotension (blood pressure 120/80 mmHg in the supine position and 80/60 mmHg upon standing). Neurological examinations revealed weakness, atrophy (Fig. 3.6), and generalized areflexia in the four extremities. Muscle power examination revealed normal or weakness of the following muscle group: neck flexion, Medical Research Council (MRC) grade 5/5; shoulder

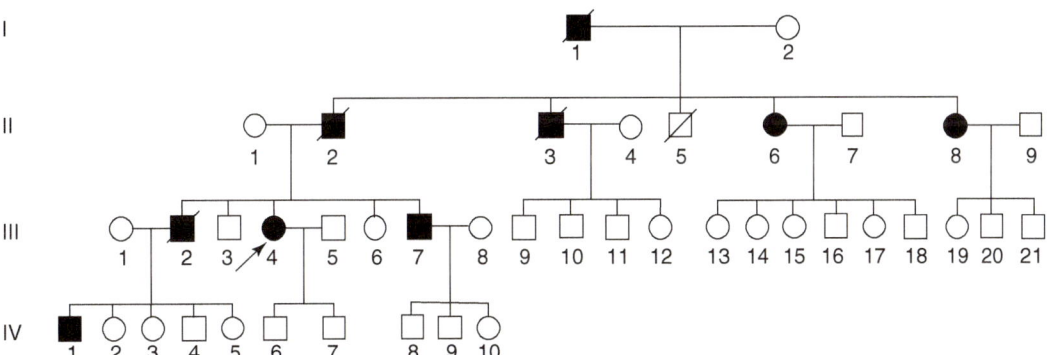

Fig. 3.5 The family pedigree of the patient. *Square* indicates male; *circle*, females; *empty symbol*, unaffected individual; *filled symbol*, affected individual; *arrow*, proband; *diagonal line* across symbol, deceased individual. I_1 died at age 65 with symptoms of FAP since age of 60. II_2 died at age 54 with symptoms of FAP since age 45. III_2 died at age 52

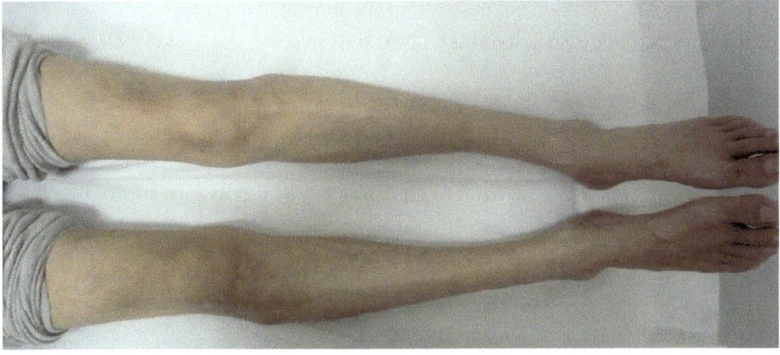

Fig. 3.6 Lower limbs muscle atrophy of the patient. The lower part of legs looks like "stork legs" or "inverted champagne bottle"

abduction, MRC grade 4/5; wrist flexion and extension, MRC grade 3/5; hip flexion, MRC grade 3/5; ankle flexion and extension, MRC grade 2/5. Sensation examination revealed pinprick and temperature sensations were absent, and vibration and proprioception sensations were decreased. Babinski sign was negative.

The patient had normal laboratory studies, including full blood count, blood biochemical tests, vitamin B12 and folate levels, thyroid function tests, parathyroid and testosterone hormone levels, and autoantibodies and paraneoplastic antibodies test. Nerve conduction studies displayed normal motor nerve conduction but reduced sensory nerve action potential (SNAP) in the upper limbs and absent SNAP and reduced compound muscle action potentials (CMAP) in the lower limbs, suggestive of a distal axonal neuropathy or length-dependent, axonal type sensorimotor peripheral neuropathy. Ophthalmoscope after pupil dilation and eye ultrasound revealed vitreous opacity in bilateral side.

Primary Diagnosis

Progressive paresthesia and weakness in four extremities as the main features of this patient, reduced muscle power, decreased superficial and deep sensation and generalized areflexia in neurological examinations, and abnormal results in nerve conduction study suggest the impairment of peripheral nervous system. Orthostatic hypotension, dry skin, and skin ulcer suggest autonomic nervous system involvement. Visual problem and vitreous opacity in ophthalmoscope and eye ultrasound examination suggest extra-nervous system involvement. Level diagnosis was thus located in peripheral nervous system, autonomic nervous system, and extra-nervous system. Based on the autosomal-dominant inheritance of her family, hereditary motor and sensory neuropathy should be considered. However, the rapid progress course did not support this disease. Combined with obvious autonomic dysfunction and vitreous opacity, familial amyloid polyneuropathy (FAP) should be considered. In the three main types of FAP, transthyretin-related FAP (TTR-FAP) and apolipoprotein A-1 FAP could cause a nerve length-dependent polyneuropathy. But the length-dependent polyneuropathy is not the predominant feature of apolipoprotein A-1 FAP, which induced the major organ damage preferably. Therefore, TTR-FAP could be the first diagnosis. To make it clear, nerve biopsy and genetic screening of *TTR* gene should be conducted.

Additional Tests or Key Results

Biopsy of sural nerve showed the presence of extracellular amyloid deposits in the endoneurial space, which confirmed our hypothesis (Fig. 3.7). The entire coding sequence and the exon/intron boundaries of *TTR* gene were sequencing. Mutation c.145A>G (p.T49A) were detected in the patient and his affected relatives, which had been reported as deleteriously before (Fig. 3.8). This result further confirmed the diagnosis of FAP.

Discussion

TTR-FAP is an autosomal-dominant inherited disease related to mutations within the *TTR* gene. The mutations in *TTR* result in misfolding of the protein and the formation of amyloid fibrils. Insoluble amyloid fibrils can deposit in multiple organs and tissues, which leads to sensorimotor neuropathy, autonomic neuropathy, cardiomyopa-

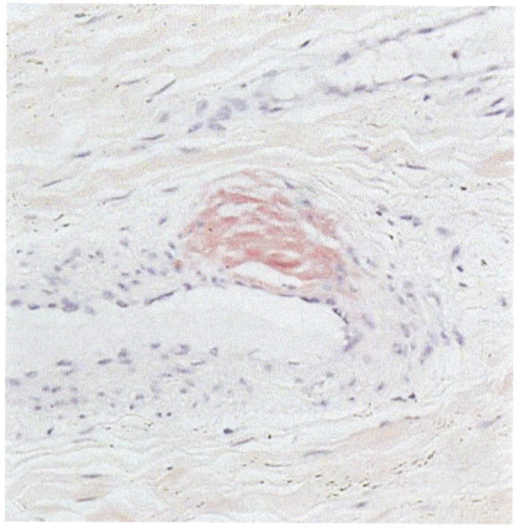

Fig. 3.7 Sural nerve biopsy from the patient. Congo red staining verifies the presence of amyloid in the endoneurium and around an endoneurial vessel

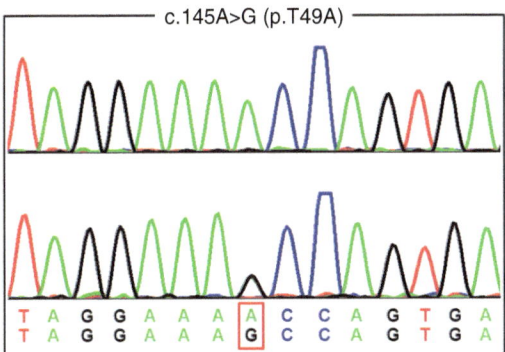

c.145A>G (p.T49A)

| T | A | G | G | A | A | A | A | C | C | A | G | T | G | A |
| T | A | G | G | A | A | A | G | C | C | A | G | T | G | A |

Fig. 3.8 Chromatogram of the heterozygous c.145A>G (p.T49A) mutation within *TTR* gene

thy, nephropathy, leptomeningeal amyloidosis, and vitreous opacities [33]. A wide clinical spectrum and considerable phenotypic heterogeneities make the diagnosis challenging. Therefore, many patients lose therapeutic opportunities, and the median survival time is about 10 years in endemic areas, even shorter in other places [34]. TTR-FAP is often fetal, devastating, and irreversible.

As in this patient, length-dependent sensorimotor axonal polyneuropathy is the typical peripheral nerve deficit trait of FAP. It is firstly involved in unmyelinated nerve fibers, then small myelinated nerve fibers, and large myelinated nerve fibers. Clinically, neurological deficits progress in a direction from feet to ankle, lower leg, thigh, fingers, fore arm, and anterior trunk. Generally, symptoms start with impaired pain and thermal sensation, followed by abnormality of light touch, deep sensation, and motor fiber deficits. So numbness and pain of the feet should be the first sign, which usually is neglected by the patients and their doctors. Other than that, it can't be detected by the routine conduction studies.

TTR-FAP should be considered highly, if a patient has a positive family history, length-dependent sensorimotor axonal polyneuropathy, and symptoms of amyloid deposits in extra-neurological organs. However, some patients present as sporadic TTR-FAP because of late onset and low penetrance. These patients should differentiate with CIDP because of high CSF protein level, differentiate with diabetic polyneuropathy because of length-dependent sensorimotor polyneuropathy or early small fiber deficit, and differentiate with toxic neuropathy because of axonal neuropathy. In a previous study, 18 in 90 nonfamilial cases were misdiagnosed and treated as CIDP [35]. For these intractable cases, nerve biopsy and *TTR* gene screening is mandatory to make a differential diagnosis.

For the patients with TTR-FAP, symptomatic treatments are necessary and can provide immediate relief, such as treating neuroglia with gabapentin, treating gastroparesis with domperidone, and treating vitreous opacity with vitrectomy [36]. However, the key to treatment is to stop the successive amyloid deposition. In this file, the liver transplantation is the standardized treatment strategy, which could eliminate the production of the mutant TTR and halt the polyneuropathy progression. But the liver transplantation has no effect to cardiomyopathy and ocular amyloidosis and need to be done in the early course of FAP [37]. Otherwise, TTR stabilizer tafamidis, which was approved by European medical agency, is another option for the patients in the early stage [38]. Gene therapies also show great promise [36]. But patients in the current study were complicated with severe motor deficits when they were diagnosed, and all the modifying treatments were not eligible.

3.5   Charcot-Marie-Tooth Disease (CMT)

A 39-Year-Old Male with Leg Weakness and Kyphoscoliosis

Clinical Presentations

A 39-year-old Chinese man presented with one year history of bilateral distal leg weakness. Over the previous year, it was difficult for him to climb the stairs. He always experienced slippers fall off when walking over uneven surfaces. He found his both legs were progressively becoming thinner. The symptoms did not show a fluctuating course. There was no history of joint pain, numbness, headache, cognitive problems, hearing impairment, eyelid drooping, swallowing difficulty, or shortness of breath. He said he was not a good runner and was unable to keep up with his peers during childhood. Since he was 10 years old, his parents noticed that he had kyphoscoliosis. He had no other medical problems and was not taking any medications. No family history of neurologic disease was recorded (Fig. 3.9a).

Neurological examinations showed symmetrical weakness of ankle dorsiflexion (Medical Research Council [MRC] grade 4/5) in the lower extremity. He had moderate atrophy of distal muscle of the lower limbs. Tendon reflex in all limbs were absent. He also had claw hands, pes cavus with hammer toes, and kyphoscoliosis (Fig. 3.9b). The sensation of pinprick and vibration were reduced below both knees. The hand and the foot were cold and wet. Cognition, cranial nerves, and cerebellar functions were normal. No pathological reflexes were found.

The laboratorial studies revealed that the C-reactive protein, erythrocyte sedimentation rate, creatine kinase, vitamin B12, folate, thyroid function, immunoglobulins, and electrolytes

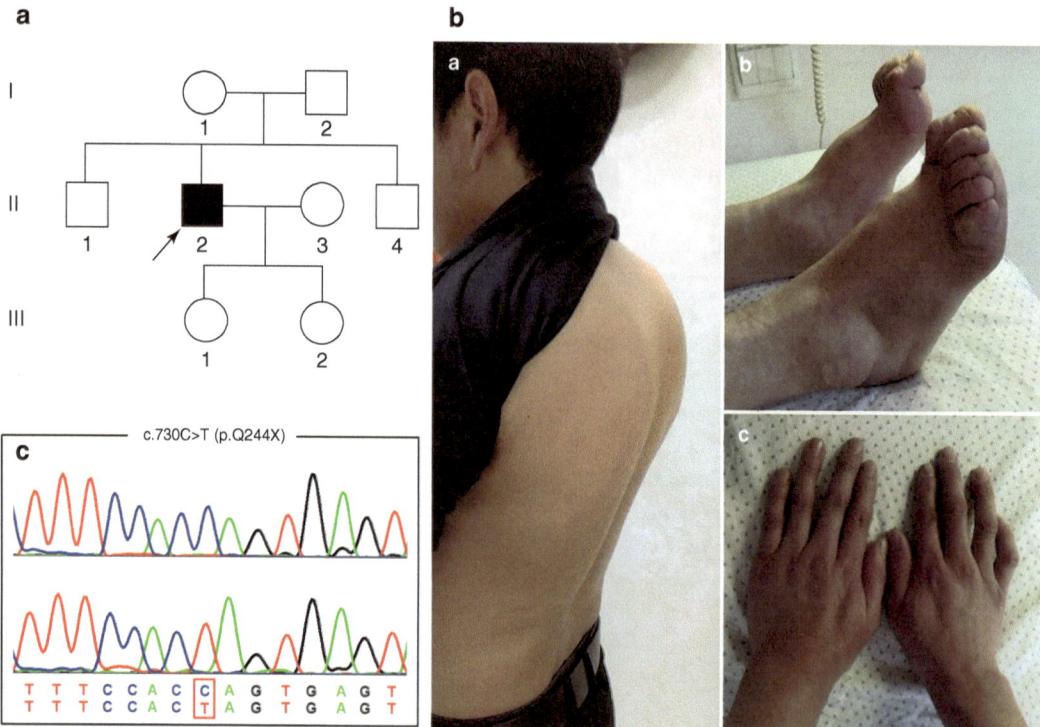

Fig. 3.9 The pedigree, clinical manifestation, and sequencing analyses of the patient. (**a**) Pedigree of the patient. The index is indicated by the *arrow*. The *black box* indicates the affected patient. (**b**) Clinical manifestation of the patient: scoliosis (*a*), foot deformity (*b*), and claw hand (*c*). (**c**) The sequencing chromatograms showing a homozygous variant in *SH3TC2*. The substitution (C > T) at base 730 results in a stop signal (TAG) at codon 244 (p.Q244X) in *SH3TC2*

were all within normal range. Serology for HIV, hepatitis, and syphilis were negative. The antineutrophil cytoplasmic and antinuclear antibodies were also negative.

Primary Diagnosis

The signs of symmetrical distal motor weakness, generalized areflexia, sensation impairment in a distal stocking pattern, and negative Babinski sign hint the involvement of peripheral nerves. Diseases that affect the peripheral nerves should be differentiated, such as chronic acquired neuropathies and inherited polyneuropathy. Diabetes is one of the most common causes of neuropathy, but our patient did not suffer from this problem. Moreover, no history of toxic contact and nutritional deficiency was reported. Systemic diseases like POEMS syndrome (polyneuropathy, organomegaly, endocrinopathy, monoclonal gammopathy, skin changes) and systemic lupus erythematosus (SLE) exhibit symptoms of peripheral nerve involvement. Nevertheless, only a negligible number of patients display polyneuropathy before advanced stages of the disease. In our patient, the positive antinuclear antibodies, hepatomegaly, and skin changes were not observed. Hence, we did not consider these systemic diseases.

Further electrophysiological studies were necessary to confirm the deficit of peripheral nerves. Lumbar puncture with cerebrospinal fluid (CSF) analysis was required to exclude the chronic acquired neuropathies, such as chronic inflammatory demyelinating polyneuropathy (CIDP).

Additional Tests or Key Results

CSF analysis showed normal protein and cell counts. The IgG-oligoclonal bands were present in both CSF and serum. Electrophysiological examination revealed decreased motor nerve conduction velocities (MNCV) and absent sensory nerve action potentials (SNAP) in the tested nerves (Table 3.2).

According to the electrophysiological study, we can verify the impairment of peripheral nerves. The CSF examination is normal, helping to differentiate it from CIDP. The following characteristics of this patient may point to genetic neurological disorders: early age of onset, slowly progressive disease course, widespread slowing of conduction velocities, and presence of pes cavus and scoliosis. The differential diagnosis for inherited polyneuropathies includes Charcot-Marie-Tooth (CMT), familial amyloid polyneuropathy (FAP), Refsum's disease, and porphyric neuropathy.

FAP is featured by the predominant involvement of small diameter sensory and autonomic nerves and deposition of amyloid in various organs. The pattern of inheritance in all types is autosomal dominant. Sensory loss, pain, and autonomic changes are prominent in the disease. Cardiac enlargement and irregularities in cardiac rhythm have occurred in most patients. The diagnosis of Refsum's disease is based on a

Table 3.2 Electrophysiological study of the patient

Motor nerve conduction study								
	Median		Ulnar		Peroneal		Tibial	
Nerve	Right	Left	Right	Left	Right	Left	Right	Left
MNCV (m/s)	31	30	29	27	18	13	25	19
CMAP (mV)	4.484	8.323	6.270	6.849	0.336	0.083	0.550	0.771
Sensor nerve conduction study								
	Median		Ulnar		Radial		Sural	
Nerve	Right	Left	Right	Left	Right	Left	Right	Left
SNCV (m/s)	NP	NP	NP	NP	NP	NP	NP	NP
SNAP (μV)	NP	NP	NP	NP	NP	NP	NP	NP

MNCV motor nerve conduction velocity, *CMAP* compound motor action potential, *SNCV* sensory nerve conduction velocity, *SNAP* sensory nerve action potential, *NP* not potential

combination of clinical manifestations including retinitis pigmentosa, ataxia, and chronic polyneuropathy. Cardiomyopathy and neurogenic deafness are present in most patients. The most characteristics of porphyric neuropathy are the relapsing nature, acute onset, abdominal pain, psychotic symptoms, and predominant motor neuropathy. In our patient, normal color Doppler echocardiography and ECG examination were reported. Some typical symptoms, such as cardiac enlargement, ataxia, and abdominal pain, were not observed. Consequently, we did not primarily consider these inherited diseases.

Since CMT is the most common disease responsible for the inherited polyneuropathy, we pay our attention to this disease. The MNCV of the examined nerve was significantly decreased indicated the demyelinating type of CMT. As *PMP22* duplication/deletion was the major genetic cause for demyelinating CMT, we first carried out multiplex ligation-dependent probe amplification (MLPA) analysis to detect the copy number of *PMP22*. However, the result was negative. To make sure the causative gene responsible for this patient, we designed a gene panel covering 70 genes associated with CMT (Table 3.3). Then the targeted next-generation

sequencing (NGS) was performed. After filtering, a homozygous variant (c.730C>T) caused a premature SH3TC2 protein (p.Q244X) was observed in the *SH3TC2* gene. This variant was verified by Sanger sequencing (Fig. 3.9c) and was not present in our 500 controls. On the basis of the American College of Medical Genetic and Genomics (ACMG) standard and guideline, this novel variant in *SH3TC2* was classified as pathogenicity [39]. Thus, the patient was finally diagnosed with CMT. Pathological examination was not tested as the patient refused nerve biopsy.

Discussion

CMT, also known as hereditary motor and sensory neuropathy, is the most common hereditary neuromuscular disorder. It is clinically characterized by progressive motor weakness and sensory abnormalities. The incidence of CMT was evaluated up to 1 in 2500 people. In light of the nerve conduction studies, CMT could be subdivided into three main groups: a demyelinating form (MNCV <38 m/s; CMT1 if autosomal dominant), an axonal form, and an intermediate form (MNCV lies between 25 and 45 m/s). Further subdivision of these CMT types is based mainly on causative genes [40]. All Mendelian inheritance modes are

Table 3.3 List of genes responsible for CMT and other hereditary peripheral neuropathy

No.	Gene	No.	Gene	No.	Gene	No.	Gene
1	AARS	19	INF2	37	RAB7B	55	DST
2	BSCL2	20	KARS	38	SBF1	56	FAM134B
3	CCT5	21	KIF1B	39	SBF2	57	HSN1B
4	CTDP1	22	LITAF	40	SEPT9	58	IKBKAP
5	DHTKD1	23	LMNA	41	SH3TC2	59	KIF1A
6	DNM2	24	LRSAM1	42	SOX10	60	NGF
7	DYNC1H1	25	MED25	43	SURF1	61	NTRK1
8	EGR2	26	MFN2	44	TRPV4	62	SCN11A
9	FGD4	27	MPZ	45	YARS	63	SPTLC1
10	FIG4	28	MTMR2	46	DCTN1	64	SPTLC2
11	GARS	29	NDRG1	47	FBXO38	65	WNK1
12	GDAP1	30	NEFL	48	HSPB3	66	ALAD
13	GJB1	31	PDK3	49	IGHMBP2	67	CPOX
14	GNB4	32	PLEKHG5	50	REEP1	68	HMBS
15	HK1	33	PMP22	51	SLC5A7	69	PPOX
16	HOXD10	34	PRPS1	52	ATL1	70	TTR
17	HSPB1	35	PRX	53	ATL3		
18	HSPB8	36	RAB7A	54	DNMT1		

described for CMT, and over 50 causative genes have been described to be related with CMT (http://www.molgen.ua.ac.be/CMTMutations/; http://neuromuscular.wustl.edu/).

The genetic diagnosis of CMT patient was performed according to the inheritance pattern, clinical phenotype, and neurophysiologic results. Our patient displayed a demyelinating form of CMT without positive family history. As *PMP22* is the most causative gene [41], the *PMP22* duplication/deletion analysis should be investigated first in patient with autosomal-dominant or sporadic demyelinating form of CMT.

Using targeted NGS, we identified a homozygous variant in *SH3TC2* in our patient. *SH3TC2* is the causative gene responsible for CMT type 4C (CMT4C) [42]. Both missense and nonsense mutations in the gene have been reported [43]. CMT4C is an autosomal-recessive demyelinating form of CMT. It is clinically manifested by early-onset demyelinating peripheral neuropathy frequently associated with spinal deformities and cranial nerves involvement. In the first decade of life, the CMT4C patient usually has severe spine deformities, such as scoliosis or kyphoscoliosis [44–46]. The progress of spine deformities is usually faster than motor deficits. Our patient showed slowly progressive motor impairments but had early onset of spinal deformities. In addition, the symptoms of cranial nerves deficits, such as hearing loss, dysphagia, diplopia, and vocal cord paresis, are found in most CMT4C cases [45]. However, our patient did not show these symptoms. Nerve biopsy is an effective approach to observe the myelin abnormalities in CMT4C patients.

Currently, there is no effective pharmacologic therapy for CMT. Fortunately, CMT4C patient shows a slowly progressive course. The treatment objectives for CMT are to enhance the quality of life and reduce deformities. Patients with CMT should be avoiding taking drugs that cause peripheral nerve toxicity. A series of trials using ascorbic acid for CMT1A has been carried out; however, these trails failed to show any benefit to CMT1A patients [47]. Many different approaches have been used to treat feet and spine deformities, including rehabilitative therapy and surgical treatment [40]. Surgery was required when the scoliosis cause respiratory difficulties. Genetic counseling for patients and their families is important.

3.6 Charcot-Marie-Tooth Disease Plus Acute Inflammatory Demyelinating Polyradiculoneuropathy (CMT + AIDP)

A 29-Year-Old Male with a More Than 20-Years History of Unsteadiness and Aggravated for One Month

Clinical Presentations

Mr. Xu is a 29-year-old shopkeeper who presented to us with a more than 20-years history of unsteady on his feet. He had noticed "heaviness" in his feet since he was a toddler and was easy to stumble while running. His symptoms progressed gradually very slow that did not affect his daily life until last month. His walking has deteriorated rapidly since last month, and he has to put a lot of effort to lift his feet, as if he is "walking with concrete blocks on," particularly while walking upstairs.

On examination, Mr. Xu's general systemic examinations, including pulse and blood pressure, were unremarkable. The cranial nerves were normal. Symmetrical distal atrophy was found in the hands and in the legs to knees level. Muscle tone was normal. Power examination revealed symmetrical weakness in the feet (MRC grade: 3/5) and throughout the hands (MRC grade: 4/5). Deep sensation including joint position sense and vibration sense were decreased in the legs to knee level, while light touch sensation and pain sensation were not impaired. Ankle and knee reflexes were absent, and other reflexes were decreased.

Primary Diagnosis

The history and examination findings suggested that there was a combination of sensory and motor symptoms, affecting the distal of all four limbs. Nerve conduction study revealed widespread slowing of conduction velocity in sensory and motor nerves, as shown in Table 3.4. This could be compatible with a length-dependent peripheral nerve disorder. Because of the early onset and very long history, hereditary peripheral neuropathy would be the first consideration, of which Charcot-Marie-Tooth disease (CMT) is most frequent. On further query, Mr. Xu reported that his father and uncle's legs seem to be thinner than normal, but there was no muscle weakness. This family history also argued in favor of the diagnosis of CMT.

Additional Tests or Key Results

However, the CSF analysis indicated an elevated protein level of 1.02 g/L (0.1–0.45 g/L). This increased protein level would not be produced by CMT, which always has a normal or slightly elevated protein level. At this point, we had to go back to our history collection. Did

Table 3.4 Nerve conduction study

Nerve	Stimulate point	Latency (ms)	Amplitude (mV)	Velocity (m/s)
Motor nerve conduction velocity (MNCV)				
Ulnar (R)	Wrist	9.5	2.4	
	Elbow	24.1	1.6	14.3
Median (R)	Wrist	14.7	3.0	
	Elbow	29.9	2.0	13.5
Peroneus (R)	Ankle	23.3	0.5	
	Capitula fibula	41.3	0.5	13.9
Tibial (R)	Medial malleolus	21.0	0.4	
	Popliteal fossa	51.2	0.3	11.6
Sensory nerve conduction velocity (SNCV)				
Superficial ulnar (R)	Pinkie	3.0	2.7	34.5
Superficial median (R)	Middle finger	3.7	1.4	35.1
Sural (R)	14 cm above heel	2.8	0.9	24.7
Superficial peroneus (R)	One third of leg	2.8	0.2	35.7

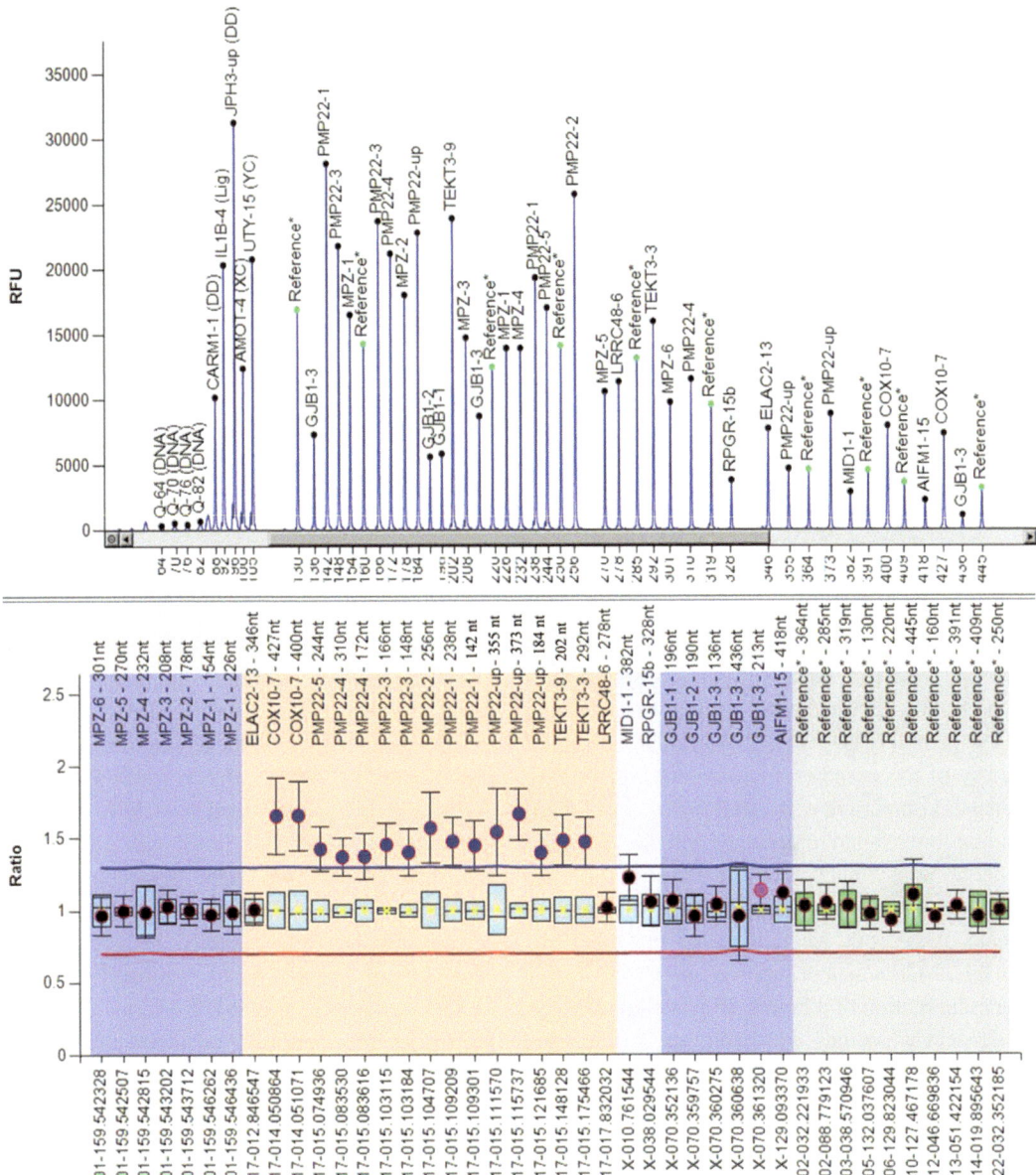

Fig. 3.10 Multiplex ligation-dependent probe amplification (MLPA) revealed the abnormal duplication of *PMP22* gene

Mr. Xu really have a 20-year disease history? Was the family history reliable? Was it possible that his unsteadiness only developed for the latest month and the long disease duration as well as the family history was our misleading? If there was only one month's history, the diagnosis of acute inflammatory demyelinating polyradiculoneuropathy (AIDP) should be in the first order. However, the symmetrical distal atrophy of the limbs could not be explained by a one-month history.

PMP22 genotyping was requested and was positive (Fig. 3.10), which confirmed the diagnosis of CMT1A. However, did this mean that the disorder of CMT could cause an elevated CSF protein level? We revealed the relevant papers

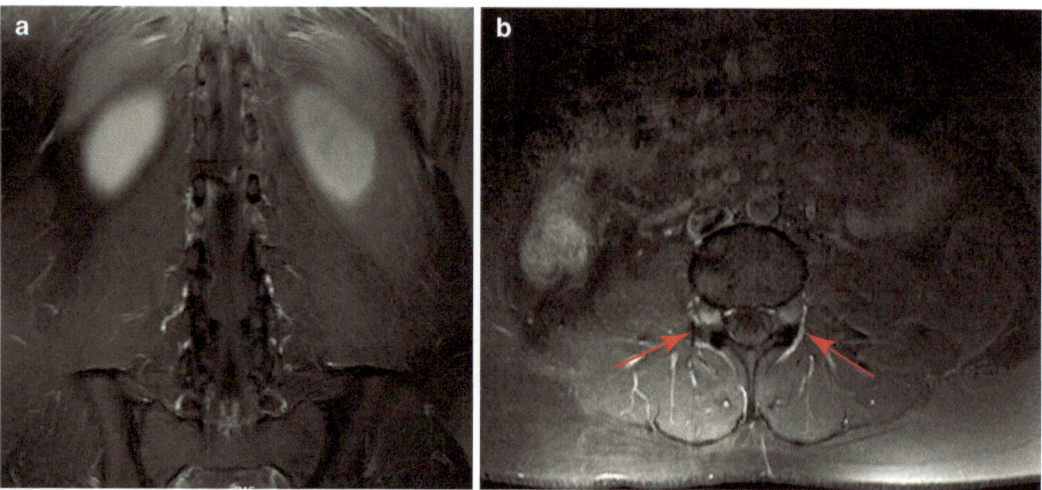

Fig. 3.11 MRI of the lumbosacral spine, coronal (**a**) and axial (**b**). T2-weighted images show thickened nerve roots that completely fill the dural sac. In (**b**), the *red arrow* heads indicate the hypertrophic ganglia

and found a few case reports of this phenomenon [48–51]. Most of these patients presented with hypertrophy of spinal roots, which was also seen in our patient (Fig. 3.11). Some researchers did a biopsy of the peripheral nerve, and a pathology that was compatible with AIDP/CIDP was found. Although we failed to persuade Mr. Xu to receive a nerve biopsy, his symptoms did alleviate a lot after the administration of steroids for several weeks. As a result, we hypothesize that there was an AIDP/CIDP superimposed on CMT1A, for the combination of a high CSF protein level with the recent worsening. However, we were unable to differentiate AIDP from CIDP because there was no confirmatory evidence in laboratory or morphologic findings.

Discussion

This patient showed chronic motor-sensory poly-neuropathy since childhood and acute symptoms worsening for one month. His history and labora-tory findings suggested AIDP/CIDP overlapping CMT1A. Both AIDP/CIDP and CMT have the distal muscle weakness and areflexia. However, in this case, the patient's early age of onset, the presence of muscle atrophy in lower limbs, and deformities were explained by CMT. Although the patient's inheritance mode was not clear, it suggested an autosomal dominance trait.

The occurrence of CMT1A overlapping with AIDP/CIDP has been reported in several cases. Most of them were genetically confirmed and all had an increased protein level in CSF. Besides, hypertro-phy of spinal roots was also an important character.

Although CMT is a neural hereditary disease that with no effective therapy at present, AIDP/ CIDP is a gained disorder that respond well to IVIG or glucocorticoid. As a result, we suggest that the phenomenon seen in our case should be recognized, and targeted therapy should be started up as early as possible to prevent the development of the disease.

3.7 Kennedy's Disease

A 51-Year-Old Male with Weakness of Limbs and Atrophy of Tongue

Clinical Presentations

A 51-year-old man visited our clinic for one-year difficulty of climbing stairs and weakness of holding stuffs. He also reported a progressively developing swallowing problem and a slurred speech within 3 months. He denied any seizures, vertigo, blurred vision, memory loss, and sensory abnormalities. Besides, he reported no recent illness, sick contacts, or travel abroad and family history of neuromuscular disorders.

On neurological examinations, his vital signs were notable for an obvious atrophy of tongue muscle, weakness of neck muscle, and mild to moderate atrophy and weakness of limb muscles. His strength of both proximal upper limbs was 4/5 per Medical Research Council (MRC) scale; strength of both distal upper limbs was 5−/5 per MRC scale. His strength of both proximal lower limbs was 3/5, and strength of distal lower limbs was 4/5. The patient's bilateral tendon reflexes were decreased. Sensation was grossly intact. The rest neurological examinations were normal apart from his breast development (gynecomastia).

His cervical MRI revealed slightly bulging of disk C3/4 and C6/7. Blood tests revealed a significantly elevated creatine kinase (CK) up to 672 U/L (reference range 38–174 U/L) and a slightly elevated lactate dehydrogenase (LDH). The rest imaging and lab tests including cerebrospinal fluid (CSF) tests were all negative.

Primary Diagnosis

The patient's weakness and atrophy of multiple muscles might hint the involvement of upper motor neuron, lower motor neuron, muscles, or peripheral nerves. The decreased tendon reflex and absence of pyramidal signs further narrowed the localization to lower motor neuron, muscles, and peripheral nerves. The atrophy of tongue muscle is more likely to be found in motor neuron disease (MND). However, the patient was a middle-aged male while displaying unusual breast development. Thus, a diagnosis of X-linked recessive spinal and bulbar muscular atrophy (SBMA) was strongly hinted. Meanwhile, other pure lower motor neuron disorders like spinal muscular atrophy (SMA) and peripheral nerve disorders especially acquired diseases including diabetic peripheral neuropathy (DPN) and chronic inflammatory demyelinating polyneuropathies (CIDP) might not be excluded. Additionally, considering patient's mild elevated serum CK, late-onset recessive inherited muscle disorders including some types of limb girdle muscular dystrophy (LGMD) might not be excluded either. Besides, in some stages of amyotrophic lateral sclerosis (ALS), patient's sign of upper motor neuron involvement might be absent. More precise diagnosis should rely on neurophysiological studies.

Additional Tests or Key Results

Electromyography (EMG) examination and nerve conduction study (NCS) were then carried out in this patient. The results are listed below (Table 3.5). The neurophysiological tests revealed a sporadic anterior spinal cord neuron involvement. However, the amplitude of sensory nerve action potential (SNAP) in sural nerve was also obviously decreased, hinted an involvement of sensory neuron or sensory nerve axon. The neurophysiological studies ruled out the possibilities of muscle and peripheral nerve diseases and narrowed down the diagnosis to motor neuron diseases. The involvement of sensory nerve is much more common in SBMA rather than ALS. Additional hormone tests and gene test for *AR* gene were further performed. The hormone tests demonstrated a significantly elevated serum estradiol (196.9 pmol/L, reference range in male: 28–156 pmol/L). The Sanger sequencing of the first exon of *AR* gene revealed a prolonged CAG expansion (52 repeats, Fig. 3.12).

Discussion

SBMA, also known as Kennedy's disease, is an X-linked recessive neurodegenerative disease. It's clinically characterized by slowly progressive weakness and atrophy of bulbar and proximal limbs muscles [52]. It is related to a prolonged

Table 3.5 Electromyography (EMG) and nerve conduction study (NCS) tests

Electromyography (EMG)

Muscles (right)	Insertion potential	Spontaneous potentials			MUP	Recruitment order
		Fibrillation	Positive sharp wave	Fasciculation		
Tibialis anterior	N	1+	1+	N	>5 mV	Simple
Gastrocnemius caput medialis	N	N	1+	N	>5 mV	Simple
Vastus medialis	N	N	N	N	>5 mV	Simple
Interosseus dorsal I	N	N	1+	N	>5 mV	Simple
Flexor carpi radialis	N	N	N	N	>5 mV	Simple
Biceps	N	N	1+	N	>5 mV	Simple
Rectus abdominis	N	N	N	N	>5 mV	Simple
Trapezius	N	N	1+	N	>5 mV	Simple
Sternocleidomastoid	N	N	N	N	>5 mV	Simple
Glossus	N	N	N	N	Slightly abnormal	Simple-mixed
Masseter	N	N	N	N	Slightly abnormal	Interference

Nerve conduction study (NCS)

Motor (right)	Latency (ms)	Amplitude (mV)	Distance (mm)	Velocity (m/s)	F-wave latency (ms)	
Median						
Wrist-APB	3.0	5.3	48		25.3	
Elbow-wrist	7.1	4.6	235	57.3		
Ulnar						
Wrist-ADM	3.3	8.6	53		27.9	
Below elbow-wrist	6.7	7.8	204	60.0		
Above elbow-below elbow	9.0	6.4	100	58.8		
Peroneal						
Ankle-EDB	4.4	0.8	60		NP	
Below knee-ankle	10.9	0.7	312	48.0		
Above knee-below knee	13.2	0.6	95	41.3		
Sensory (right)		Latency (ms)	Amplitude (mV)	Distance (mm)	Velocity (m/s)	
Median	Digitus III-wrist	2.4	30	128	68.1	
Ulnar	Digitus V-wrist	2.2	13	112	69.1	
Sural	Middle lower leg- lateral malleolus	2.9	2.2	120	52.2	

ADM abductor digiti minimi, *APB* abductor pollicis brevis, *EDB* extensor digitorum brevis, *NP* no potential

expansion of CAG repeats within exon 1 of androgen receptor (*AR*) gene on the X chromosome [53]. The European Federation of the Neurological Societies (EFNS) guideline indicated that an expansion beyond 38 repeats is pathogenic [54].

Even though SBMA is an inherited disorder, the report of family history remains uncommon in China [55]. In this case, the patient didn't recall any family history as well, which made the diagnosis of SBMA more difficult. The involvement of anterior spinal cord is a shared feature both in ALS and SBMA, which might easily lead to a misdiagnosis.

However, SBMA displays its identical features. Firstly, the progression of SBMA tends to

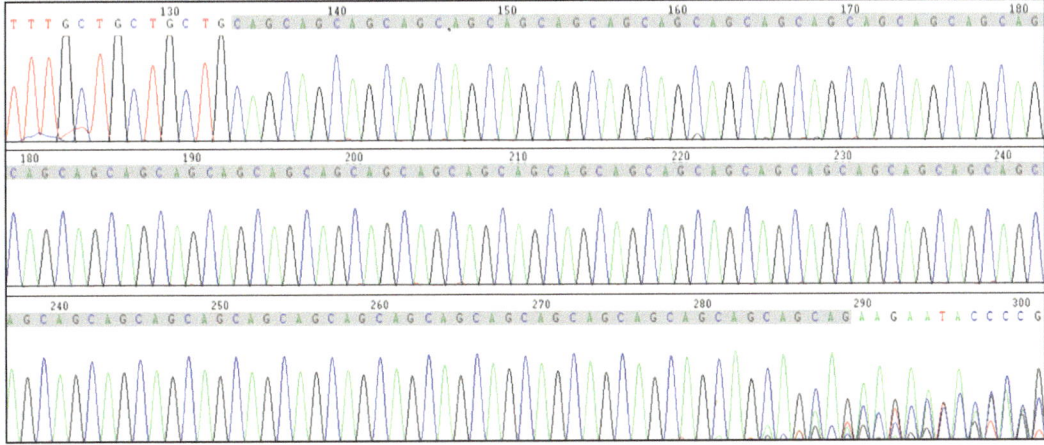

Fig. 3.12 Sequencing chromatogram of the expanded CAG repeats within *AR* in the index patient. The sequence highlighted with *gray* indicates expanded allele with 52 CAG repeats

be much slower. Patients suffered from SBMA usually live relatively long life before disabled. Moreover, it is not rare to identify muscles involvement in SBMA patients, since the expanded and misfolded polyglutamines can be seen everywhere in human body including muscles. Thus, it has been reported frequently that the serum CK in SBMA patients usually elevated [55–58]. The most important feature of SBMA is the reduction of SNAP amplitude in NCS tests. As was reported before, the reduction of SNAP amplitude can be recognized in most SBMA patients, especially in lower limbs [55, 57], which differ from ALS [59]. In this case, the patient's neurophysiological tests revealed a significantly decreased sural SNAP, which lead to further hormone and gene tests for SBMA.

Although no effective treatments have been established in SBMA so far, a few clinical trials have been accomplished. For instance, leuprorelin is a potent luteinizing hormone-releasing hormone (LHRH) analog which suppresses the release of gonadotrophins and reduces the level of testosterone generated by the testes. In 2003, Kasuno et al. [60] reported its improvement of motor function in SBMA transgenic mice. Later in 2010, a randomized and multicenter trial about leuprorelin treatment in SBMA patients was performed. Though the primary endpoint outcomes of this clinical trial failed to show efficacy, it did show improved

swallowing function in patients with disease duration less than 10 years, suggesting that the disease duration might have influenced the results [61]. Additionally, the dutasteride trial conducted by Fernández-Rhodes and colleagues failed to prove an efficacy in the treatment of SBMA [62]. The clenbuterol trial found a significant improvement of mean 6-min walk test and forced vital capacity values, but the changes of outcome measures were not significantly different (e.g., ALSFRS-R scale) [63]. Indisputably, the understanding of the pathogenesis in SBMA is remarkably strong; the translation of mechanism into clinical application remains unsatisfactory. There's still a long way to go.

References

1. Brooks BR, Miller RG, Swash M, Munsat TL; World Federation of Neurology Research Group on Motor Neuron Diseases. El Escorial revisited: revised criteria for the diagnosis of amyotrophic lateral sclerosis. Amyotroph Lateral Scler Other Motor Neuron Disord. 2000;1(5):293–299.
2. Logroscino G, Traynor BJ, Hardiman O, Chiò A, Mitchell D, Swingler RJ, Millul A, Benn E, Beghi E; EURALS. Incidence of amyotrophic lateral sclerosis in Europe. J Neurol Neurosurg Psychiatry. 2010;81(4):385–390.
3. Chen S, Sayana P, Zhang X, Le W. Genetics of amyotrophic lateral sclerosis: an update. Mol Neurodegener. 2013;8:28.
4. Chesi A, Staahl BT, Jovičić A, Couthouis J, Fasolino M, Raphael AR, Yamazaki T, Elias L, Polak M, Kelly

C, Williams KL, Fifita JA, Maragakis NJ, Nicholson GA, King OD, Reed R, Crabtree GR, Blair IP, Glass JD, Gitler AD. Exome sequencing to identify de novo mutations in sporadic ALS trios. Nat Neurosci. 2013;16(7):851–855.

5. Wortmann SB, Espeel M, Almeida L, Reimer A, Bosboom D, Roels F, de Brouwer AP, Wevers RA. Inborn errors of metabolism in the biosynthesis and remodelling of phospholipids. J Inherit Metab Dis. 2015;38(1):99–110.

6. Lo Giudice T, Lombardi F, Santorelli FM, Kawarai T, Orlacchio A. Hereditary spastic paraplegia: clinical-genetic characteristics and evolving molecular mechanisms. Exp Neurol. 2014;261:518–539.

7. Magariello A, Tortorella C, Citrigno L, Patitucci A, Tortelli R, Mazzei R, Conforti FL, Ungaro C, Sproviero W, Gambardella A, Muglia M. The p.Arg416Cys mutation in SPG3a gene associated with a pure form of spastic paraplegia. Muscle Nerve. 2012;45(6):919–920.

8. de Souza PV, de Rezende Pinto WB, de Rezende Batistella GN, Bortholin T, Oliveira AS. Hereditary spastic paraplegia: clinical and genetic hallmarks. The Cerebellum. 2016;16:525–551.

9. Deluca GC, Ebers GC, Esiri MM. The extent of axonal loss in the long tracts in hereditary spastic paraplegia. Neuropathol Appl Neurobiol. 2004;30(6):576–584.

10. Finsterer J, Loscher W, Quasthoff S, Wanschitz J, Auer-Grumbach M, Stevanin G. Hereditary spastic paraplegias with autosomal dominant, recessive, X-linked, or maternal trait of inheritance. J Neurol Sci. 2012;318(1–2):1–18.

11. Li LX, Zhao SY, Liu ZJ, Ni W, Li HF, Xiao BG, Wu ZY. Improving molecular diagnosis of Chinese patients with Charcot-Marie-Tooth by targeted next-generation sequencing and functional analysis. Oncotarget. 2016; 7(19):27655–27664.

12. Zhao X, Alvarado D, Rainier S, Lemons R, Hedera P, Weber CH, Tukel T, Apak M, Heiman-Patterson T, Ming L, Bui M, Fink JK. Mutations in a newly identified GTPase gene cause autosomal dominant hereditary spastic paraplegia. Nat Genet. 2001;29(3):326–331.

13. Namekawa M, Ribai P, Nelson I, Forlani S, Fellmann F, Goizet C, Depienne C, Stevanin G, Ruberg M, Durr A, Brice A. SPG3A is the most frequent cause of hereditary spastic paraplegia with onset before age 10 years. Neurology. 2006;66(1):112–114.

14. Orlacchio A, Montieri P, Babalini C, Gaudiello F, Bernardi G, Kawarai T. Late-onset hereditary spastic paraplegia with thin corpus callosum caused by a new SPG3A mutation. J Neurol. 2011;258(7):1361–1363.

15. Durr A, Camuzat A, Colin E, Tallaksen C, Hannequin D, Coutinho P, Fontaine B, Rossi A, Gil R, Rousselle C, Ruberg M, Stevanin G, Brice A. Atlastin 1 mutations are frequent in young-onset autosomal dominant spastic paraplegia. Arch Neurol. 2004;61(12):1867–1872.

16. Ribeiro AM, Ferreira CH, Mateus-Vasconcelos ECL, Moroni RM, Brito LM, Brito LG. Physical therapy in the management of pelvic floor muscles hypertonia in a woman with hereditary spastic paraplegia. Case Rep Obstet Gynecol. 2014;2014:306028.

17. Fink JK. Hereditary spastic paraplegia: clinico-pathologic features and emerging molecular mechanisms. Acta Neuropathol. 2013;126(3):307–328.

18. Sheng-Yuan Z, Xiong F, Chen YJ, Yan TZ, Zeng J, Li L, Zhang YN, Chen WQ, Bao XH, Zhang C, Xu XM. Molecular characterization of SMN copy number derived from carrier screening and from core families with SMA in a Chinese population. Eur J Hum Genet. 2010;18(9):978–984.

19. Kolb SJ, Kissel JT. Spinal muscular atrophy: a timely review. Arch Neurol. 2011;68(8):979–984.

20. Lefebvre S, Bürglen L, Reboullet S, Clermont O, Burlet P, Viollet L, Benichou B, Cruaud C, Millasseau P, Zeviani M, Le D. Identification and characterization of a spinal muscular atrophy-determining gene. Cell. 1995;80(1):155–165.

21. Chen WJ, He J, Zhang QJ, Lin QF, Chen YF, Lin XZ, Lin MT, Murong SX, Wang N. Modification of phenotype by SMN2 copy numbers in two Chinese families with SMN1 deletion in two continuous generations. Clin Chim Acta. 2012;413(23-24):1855–1860.

22. Xu C, Chen X, Grzeschik SM, Ganta M, Wang CH. Hydroxyurea enhances SMN2 gene expression through nitric oxide release. Neurogenetics. 2011;12(1):19–24.

23. Nizzardo M, Nardini M, Ronchi D, Salani S, Donadoni C, Fortunato F, Colciago G, Falcone M, Simone C, Riboldi G, Govoni A, Bresolin N, Comi GP, Corti S. Beta-lactam antibiotic offers neuroprotection in a spinal muscular atrophy model by multiple mechanisms. Exp Neurol. 2011;229(2):214–225.

24. Naryshkin NA, Weetall M, Dakka A, Narasimhan J, Zhao X, Feng Z, Ling KK, Karp GM, Qi H, Woll MG, Chen G1, Zhang N, Gabbeta V, Vazirani P, Bhattacharyya A, Furia B, Risher N, Sheedy J, Kong R, Ma J, Turpoff A, Lee CS, Zhang X, Moon YC, Trifillis P, Welch EM, Colacino JM, Babiak J, Almstead NG, Peltz SW, Eng LA, Chen KS, Mull JL, Lynes MS, Rubin LL, Fontoura P, Santarelli L, Haehnke D, McCarthy KD, Schmucki R, Ebeling M, Sivaramakrishnan M, Ko CP, Paushkin SV, Ratni H, Gerlach I, Ghosh A, Metzger F. SMN2 splicing modifiers improve motor function and longevity in mice with spinal muscular atrophy. Science. 2014;345(6197):688–693.

25. Weihl CC, Connolly AM, Pestronk A. Valproate may improve strength and function in patients with type III/IV spinal muscle atrophy. Neurology. 2006;67(3):500–501.

26. Swoboda KJ, Scott CB, Crawford TO, Simard LR, Reyna SP, Krosschell KJ, Acsadi G, Elsheik B, Schroth MK, D'Anjou G, LaSalle B, Prior TW, Sorenson SL, Maczulski JA, Bromberg MB, Chan GM, Kissel JT; Project Cure Spinal Muscular Atrophy Investigators Network. SMA CARNI-VAL trial part I: double-blind, randomized, placebo-controlled trial of L-carnitine and valproic acid in spinal muscular atrophy. PLoS One. 2010;5(8):e12140.

27. Kissel JT, Scott CB, Reyna SP, Crawford TO, Simard LR, Krosschell KJ, Acsadi G, Elsheik B, Schroth MK, D'Anjou G, LaSalle B, Prior TW, Sorenson S, Maczulski JA, Bromberg MB, Chan GM, Swoboda KJ; Project Cure Spinal Muscular Atrophy Investigators' Network. SMA CARNIVAL TRIAL PART II: a prospective, single-armed trial of L-carnitine and valproic acid in ambulatory children with spinal muscular atrophy. PLoS One. 2011;6(7):e21296.

28. Darbar IA, Plaggert PG, Resende MB, Zanoteli E, Reed UC. Evaluation of muscle strength and motor abilities in children with type II and III spinal muscle atrophy treated with valproic acid. BMC Neurol. 2011;11:36.

29. Kissel JT, Elsheikh B, King WM, Freimer M, Scott CB, Kolb SJ, Reyna SP, Crawford TO, Simard LR, Krosschell KJ, Acsadi G, Schroth MK, D'Anjou G, LaSalle B, Prior TW, Sorenson S, Maczulski JA, Swoboda KJ; Project Cure Spinal Muscular Atrophy Investigators Network. SMA valiant trial: a prospective, double-blind, placebo-controlled trial of valproic acid in ambulatory adults with spinal muscular atrophy. Muscel Nerve. 2014;49(2):187–192.

30. Ebert AD, Yu J, Rose Jr FF, Mattis VB, Lorson CL, Thomson JA, Svendsen CN. Induced pluripotent stem cells from a spinal muscular atrophy patient. Nature. 2009;457(7227):277–280.

31. Marchetto MC, Winner B, Gage FH. Pluripotent stem cells in neurodegenerative and neurodevelopmental diseases. Hum Mol Genet. 2010;19(R1):R71–76.

32. Jang YY, Ye Z. Gene correction in patient-specific iPSCs for therapy development and disease modeling. Hum Genet. 2016;135(9):1041–1058.

33. Planté-Bordeneuve V, Said G. Familial amyloid polyneuropathy. Lancet Neurol. 2011;10(12):1086–1097.

34. Coelho T, Maurer MS, Suhr OB. THAOS-the transthyretin amyloidosis outcomes survey: initial report on clinical manifestations in patients with hereditary and wild-type transthyretin amyloidosis. Curr Med Res Opin. 2013;29(1):63–76.

35. Ikeda K, Kano O, Ito H, Kawase Y, Iwamoto K, Sato R, Sekine T, Nagata R, Nakamura Y, Hirayama T, Iwasaki Y. Diagnostic pitfalls in sporadic transthyretin familial amyloid polyneuropathy (TTR-FAP). Neurology. 2008;70(17):1576–1577.

36. Plante-Bordeneuve V. Update in the diagnosis and management of transthyretin familial amyloid polyneuropathy. J Neurol. 2014;261(6):1227–1233.

37. Yamashita T, Ando Y, Okamoto S, Misumi Y, Hirahara T, Ueda M, Obayashi K, Nakamura M, Jono H, Shono M, Asonuma K, Inomata Y, Uchino M. Long-term survival after liver transplantation in patients with familial amyloid polyneuropathy. Neurology. 2012;78(9):637–643.

38. Merkies IS. Tafamidis for transthyretin familial amyloid polyneuropathy: a randomized, controlled trial. Neurology. 2013;80(15):1444–1445.

39. Richards S, Aziz N, Bale S, Bick D, Das S, Gastier-Foster J, Grody WW, Hegde M, Lyon E, Spector E, Voelkerding K, Rehm HL, Committee

ALQA. Standards and guidelines for the interpretation of sequence variants: a joint consensus recommendation of the American College of Medical Genetics and Genomics and the Association for Molecular Pathology. Genet Med. 2015;17(5):405–424.

40. Pareyson D, Marchesi C. Diagnosis, natural history, and management of Charcot-Marie-Tooth disease. Lancet Neurol. 2009;8(7):654–667.

41. Watila MM, Balarabe SA. Molecular and clinical features of inherited neuropathies due to PMP22 duplication. J Neurol Sci. 2015;355(1–2):18–24.

42. Senderek J, Bergmann C, Stendel C, Kirfel J, Verpoorten N, De Jonghe P, Timmerman V, Chrast R, Verheijen MH, Lemke G, Battaloglu E, Parman Y, Erdem S, Tan E, Topaloglu H, Hahn A, Muller-Felber W, Rizzuto N, Fabrizi GM, Stuhrmann M, Rudnik-Schoneborn S, Zuchner S, Michael Schroder J, Buchheim E, Straub V, Klepper J, Huehne K, Rautenstrauss B, Buttner R, Nelis E, Zerres K. Mutations in a gene encoding a novel SH3/TPR domain protein cause autosomal recessive Charcot-Marie-Tooth type 4C neuropathy. Am J Hum Genet. 2003;73(5):1106–1119.

43. Lupo V, Galindo MI, Martinez-Rubio D, Sevilla T, Vilchez JJ, Palau F, Espinos C. Missense mutations in the SH3TC2 protein causing Charcot-Marie-Tooth disease type 4C affect its localization in the plasma membrane and endocytic pathway. Hum Mol Genet. 2009;18(23):4603–4614.

44. Lassuthova P, Mazanec R, Vondracek P, Siskova D, Haberlova J, Sabova J, Seeman P. High frequency of SH3TC2 mutations in Czech HMSN I patients. Clin Genet. 2011;80(4):334–345.

45. Piscosquito G, Saveri P, Magri S, Ciano C, Gandioli C, Morbin M, Di Bella D, Moroni I, Taroni FF, Pareyson D. Screening for SH3TC2 gene mutations in a series of demyelinating recessive Charcot-Marie-Tooth disease (CMT4). J Peripher Nerv Syst. 2016;21(3):142–149.

46. Azzedine H, Ravise N, Verny C, Gabreels-Festen A, Lammens M, Grid D, Vallat JM, Durosier G, Senderek J, Nouioua S, Hamadouche T, Bouhouche A, Guilbot A, Stendel C, Ruberg M, Brice A, Birouk N, Dubourg O, Tazir M, LeGuern E. Spine deformities in Charcot-Marie-Tooth 4C caused by SH3TC2 gene mutations. Neurology. 2006;67(4):602–606.

47. Micallef J, Attarian S, Dubourg O, Gonnaud PM, Hogrel JY, Stojkovic T, Bernard R, Jouve E, Pitel S, Vacherot F, Remec JF, Jomir L, Azabou E, Al-Moussawi M, Lefebvre MN, Attolini L, Yaici S, Tanesse D, Fontes M, Pouget J, Blin O. Effect of ascorbic acid in patients with Charcot-Marie-Tooth disease type 1A: a multicentre, randomised, double-blind, placebo-controlled trial. Lancet Neurol. 2009;8(12):1103–1110.

48. Liao JP, Waclawik AJ. Nerve root hypertrophy in CMT type 1A. Neurology. 2004;62(5):783.

49. Odaka M, Yuki N, Kokubun N, Hirata K, Kuwabara S. Axonal Guillain-Barre syndrome associated with axonal Charcot-Marie-Tooth disease. J Neurol Sci. 2003;211(1–2):93–97.

50. Pareyson D, Testa D, Morbin M, Erbetta A, Ciano C, Lauria G, Milani M, Taroni F. Does CMT1A

homozygosity cause more severe disease with root hypertrophy and higher CSF proteins? Neurology. 2003;60(10):1721–1722.

51. Vital A, Vital C, Lagueny A, Ferrer X, Ribiere-Bachelier C, Latour P, Petry KG. Inflammatory demyelination in a patient with CMT1A. Muscle Nerve. 2003;28(3):373–376.

52. Kennedy WR, Alter M, Sung JH. Progressive proximal spinal and bulbar muscular atrophy of late onset. A sex-linked recessive trait. Neurology. 1968;18(7): 671–680.

53. La Spada AR, Wilson EM, Lubahn DB, Harding AE, Fischbeck KH. Androgen receptor gene mutations in X-linked spinal and bulbar muscular atrophy. Nature. 1991;352(6330):77–79.

54. Burgunder JM, Schols L, Baets J, Andersen P, Gasser T, Szolnoki Z, Fontaine B, Van Broeckhoven C, Di Donato S, De Jonghe P, Lynch T, Mariotti C, Spinazzola A, Tabrizi SJ, Tallaksen C, Zeviani M, Harbo HF, Finsterer J. Efns. EFNS guidelines for the molecular diagnosis of neurogenetic disorders: motoneuron, peripheral nerve and muscle disorders. Eur J Neurol. 2011;18(2):207–217.

55. Ni W, Chen S, Qiao K, Wang N, Wu ZY. Genotype-phenotype correlation in Chinese patients with spinal and bulbar muscular atrophy. PLoS One. 2015;10(3): e0122279.

56. Atsuta N, Watanabe H, Ito M, Banno H, Suzuki K, Katsuno M, Tanaka F, Tamakoshi A, Sobue G. Natural history of spinal and bulbar muscular atrophy (SBMA): a study of 223 Japanese patients. Brain. 2006;129(Pt 6):1446–1455.

57. Rhodes LE, Freeman BK, Auh S, Kokkinis AD, La Pean A, Chen C, Lehky TJ, Shrader JA, Levy EW, Harris-Love M, Di Prospero NA, Fischbeck KH. Clinical features of spinal and bulbar muscular atrophy. Brain. 2009;132(Pt 12):3242–3251.

58. Querin G, Bertolin C, Da Re E, Volpe M, Zara G, Pegoraro E, Caretta N, Foresta C, Silvano M, Corrado D, Iafrate M, Angelini L, Sartori L, Pennuto M, Gaiani A, Bello L, Semplicini C, Pareyson D, Silani V, Ermani M, Ferlin A, Soraru G, Italian Study Group on Kennedy's Disease. Non-neural phenotype of spinal and bulbar muscular atrophy: results from a large cohort of Italian patients. J Neurol Neurosurg Psychiatry. 2015;87(8):810–816.

59. Hama T, Hirayama M, Hara T, Nakamura T, Atsuta N, Banno H, Suzuki K, Katsuno M, Tanaka F, Sobue G. Discrimination of spinal and bulbar muscular atrophy from amyotrophic lateral sclerosis using sensory nerve action potentials. Muscle Nerve. 2012;45(2):169–174.

60. Katsuno M, Adachi H, Doyu M, Minamiyama M, Sang C, Kobayashi Y, Inukai A, Sobue G. Leuprorelin rescues polyglutamine-dependent phenotypes in a transgenic mouse model of spinal and bulbar muscular atrophy. Nat Med. 2003;9(6):768–773.

61. Katsuno M, Banno H, Suzuki K, Takeuchi Y, Kawashima M, Yabe I, Sasaki H, Aoki M, Morita M, Nakano I, Kanai K, Ito S, Ishikawa K, Mizusawa H, Yamamoto T, Tsuji S, Hasegawa K, Shimohata T, Nishizawa M, Miyajima H, Kanda F, Watanabe Y, Nakashima K, Tsujino A, Yamashita T, Uchino M, Fujimoto Y, Tanaka F, Sobue G. Efficacy and safety of leuprorelin in patients with spinal and bulbar muscular atrophy (JASMITT study): a multicentre, randomised, double-blind, placebo-controlled trial. Lancet Neurol. 2010;9(9):875–884.

62. Fernandez-Rhodes LE, Kokkinis AD, White MJ, Watts CA, Auh S, Jeffries NO, Shrader JA, Lehky TJ, Li L, Ryder JE, Levy EW, Solomon BI, Harris-Love MO, La Pean A, Schindler AB, Chen C, Di Prospero NA, Fischbeck KH. Efficacy and safety of dutasteride in patients with spinal and bulbar muscular atrophy: a randomised placebo-controlled trial. Lancet Neurol. 2011;10(2):140–147.

63. Querin G, D'Ascenzo C, Peterle E, Ermani M, Bello L, Melacini P, Morandi L, Mazzini L, Silani V, Raimondi M, Mandrioli J, Romito S, Angelini C, Pegoraro E, Soraru G. Pilot trial of clenbuterol in spinal and bulbar muscular atrophy. Neurology. 2013;80(23): 2095–2098.

Movement Disorders

4

Hong-Fu Li, Yu Lin, Hao Yu, Yi Dong,
and Hong-Lei Li

Abstract

Movement disorders are a large group of diseases caused by extrapyramidal damage. Generally, movement disorders are classified into two major categories: hyperkinetic movement disorders referring to excessive, repetitive, and involuntary movements and hypokinetic movement disorders referring to akinesia, hypokinesia, bradykinesia, and rigidity. Actually, movement disorders were very common in clinical practice, with age at onset from childhood to old age. Among them, inherited movement disorders accounted for a large proportion, such as early-onset Parkinson's disease (PD), Wilson's disease (WD), Huntington's disease (HD), dopa-responsive dystonia (DRD), neuroacanthocytosis (NA), paroxysmal kinesigenic dyskinesia (PKD), pantothenate kinase-associated neurodegeneration (PKAN), and so on. Some of these disorders (such as WD, HD, PKD, etc.) have only one causative gene, while some (such as PD, DRD, NA, etc.) have more than two culprit genes. In the inherited movement disorders, neuropathology plays a less role in the diagnosis. On the contrary, detecting the disease-causing mutation is crucial for diagnosis. For example, HTT mutation is important to differentiate HD from HD-like disorders. In this chapter, we presented several movement disorders caused by genetic mutations. Some of them had typical clinical manifestations, while some are difficult to diagnose at beginning.

Keywords

Movement disorders • Parkinson's disease • Wilson's disease • Huntington's disease • Dopa-responsive dystonia • Neuroacanthocytosis • Paroxysmal kinesigenic dyskinesia • Pantothenate kinase-associated neurodegeneration

H.-F. Li (✉) • H. Yu • Y. Dong • H.-L. Li
Department of Neurology and Research Center of
Neurology, Second Affiliated Hospital, Zhejiang
University School of Medicine, Hangzhou, China
e-mail: hongfuli@zju.edu.cn

Y. Lin
Department of Neurology and Institute of Neurology,
First Affiliated Hospital, Fujian Medical University,
Fuzhou, China

4.1   Parkinson's Disease (PD)

A 22-Year-Old Male Complained About 3 Years of Limb Tremors

Clinical Presentations

The patient was a 22-year-old man who suffered limb tremors for 3 years. His developmental milestone was unremarkable until the age of 19, when he experienced intermittent tremor in left leg. This condition was aggravated in anxiety or stress but was disappeared in calmness and sleep. He did not take any medicine because he was diagnosed with anxiety neurosis in local hospital. One year later, he noticed involuntary shaking in his left hand and the flexibility of left limbs was decreased. He could not button his coat agilely when he got dressed. Amantadine was prescribed for him but was not effective enough in controlling his tremor. Oral administration of levodopa was then conducted, which significantly relieved his symptoms at low dose. In the following 1 year, he found that it was difficult to turn around. There was no fluctuation of his symptoms in the morning and afternoon. His olfactory function was not impaired, and he did not complain about unsteady gait, dysarthria, or memory impairment. The urination and defecation disturbance was not present. His younger brother had similar symptoms to him. His parents were not internuptial, and neither of them exhibited similar symptoms (Fig. 4.1).

Examination of cranial nerves revealed a clear utterance but stiff facial expression. His left hand and leg exhibited involuntary tremor at a frequency of 3–5 Hz. The muscle strength was essentially normal. Increased muscle tension was present in his four limbs. Gear-like rigidity was apparent in his left extremities. Sensory examination was unremarkable. Knee reflex was brisk bilaterally. Babinski sign was negative. Finger–nose and heel–knee–shin test could not be completed accurately.

Laboratory examinations revealed normal blood cell counting, hepatic function, vitamin B12, ceruloplasmin, serum ferritin, and thyroid hormones. Brain MRI scanning and EEG were unremarkable.

Primary Diagnosis

This was a young man with predominant feature of limb tremor. The involuntary tremor, increased muscle tension, and gear-like rigidity revealed the impairment of extrapyramidal tract. Pyramidal signs and cerebellar signs were inconspicuous in the neurological examinations. Level diagnosis was thus located in extrapyramidal tract. The early onset, progressive course of disease, and positive family history implied that this patient may have suffered from hereditary disorder. Alternatively, metabolic disturbance and intoxication should be considered too. The differential diagnosis included Wilson's disease (WD), juvenile Parkinson's disease (PD), Parkinsonism syndrome, and dopa-responsive dystonia (DRD), neurodegeneration with brain iron accumulation (NBIA), and so on. Despite autosomal recessive inheritance, WD could be excluded because of normal ceruloplasmin, hepatic function, brain MRI, and absence of Kayser–Fleisher (K-F) ring. The favorable response to levodopa and normal MRI implied that Parkinsonism syndrome was less possible. No fluctuation of his symptoms in the morning and afternoon hinted that DRD should not be listed in priority. NBIA is less common in Chinese population. Therefore, PD was the paramount consideration. Genetic screenings of autosomal recessive PD should be conducted.

Additional Tests or Key Results

Targeted next-generation sequencing including 23 PD-related genes was performed in the proband. The detected mutations were further verified by Sanger sequencing. We found two

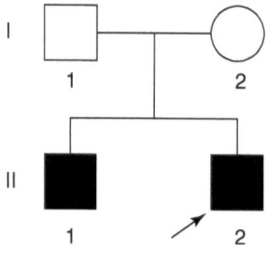

Fig. 4.1 The pedigree chart of this family. *Squares* represent males; *circles* represent females; the *black symbols* represent affected individuals; *arrows* represent the proband

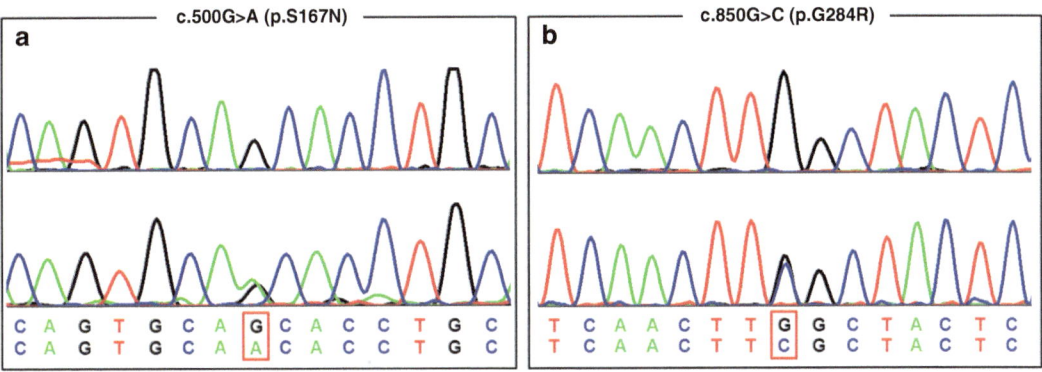

Fig. 4.2 Chromatogram of c.500G>A (**a**) and c.850G>C (**b**) mutation of *Parkin* gene. The *upper panel* depicts the normal sequence, while the *lower panel* represents heterozygous mutated sequence

compound heterozygous *Parkin* mutations, c.500G>A p.S167N and c.850G>C (p.G284R) in this patient (Fig. 4.2a, b). Further investigations revealed that his brother carried the same mutations and his father harbored p.S167N mutation and his mother carried p.G284R mutation.

Discussion

PD is the second commonest neurodegenerative disease after AD [1]. Most patients begin to exhibit symptoms after 50 years of age. However, about 10% of patients have young-onset or juvenile-onset Parkinsonism, which is generally defined as early-onset PD (EOPD) [2]. The clinical features of EOPD are not discriminative from classical PD except for the early onset [3]. Of note, the majority of EOPD cases had a positive family and harbored specific genetic mutation or variances.

The patient described here had an affected brother who had similar symptoms to him. This clearly indicated that hereditary factor should be firstly considered when we explore the etiology of his symptoms. He presented with asymmetric onset of tremor, slow progression, and favorable response to levodopa, which highly implied the diagnosis of PD. Combining the pattern of recessive inheritance,

a cluster of autosomal recessive PD gene should be screened in this patient. Using targeted NGS followed by Sanger sequencing, we detected two heterozygous Parkin mutations in this patient. The co-segregation with the disease in this family further verified that this patient was a patient of EOPD.

Parkin-linked PD has variable clinical phenotypes. Generally, most cases exhibit early-onset Parkinsonism between 30s and 40s [4]. The disease usually progresses slowly, with a favorable response to low dose of levodopa. Nevertheless, patients carrying Parkin mutation are more common to develop motor fluctuation and levodopa-induced dyskinesias during treatment [5, 6]. Cognitive impairment or dementia is rare, but behavioral problems and psychiatric symptoms have been reported with variable frequency [7, 8].

Various drugs are effective in ameliorating the PD symptoms. However, selecting the optimal treatment for PD is highly individualized. Recommending drugs for early PD consists of carbidopa/levodopa, dopamine agonists, and MAO-B inhibitors [9]. Anticholinergics, such as benzhexol, are not widely used for EOPD due to the risk of cognitive damage, confusion, hallucinations, and so on.

4.2 Paroxysmal Kinesigenic Dyskinesia (PKD)

A 17-Year-Old Male Complained About Paroxysmal Attacks of Involuntary Movements for 6 Years

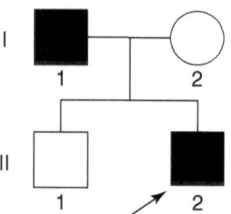

Clinical Presentations

A 17-year-old male complained about repeated transient attacks of involuntary movements for 6 years. He had an unremarkable birth and development milestone, with exception of febrile seizure from 8 months to 2 years old. At the age of 11, he developed sudden attacks of chorea which was first evident when he began to run in gym class. His arms extended and his hands flexed, followed by athetotic movement of his torso. He was aware of his attacks but could not control the episodes. The attacks usually lasted 20–40 s. A diagnosis of epilepsy was rendered in local hospital and valproate was prescribed for him. However, valproate did not show remarkable effect on relieving his attacks. In the following 3 years, he developed many such attacks which are usually triggered by sudden movement such as standing up, starting walking or running, and shifting position. The events usually lasted less than 1 min and occurred up 3–10 times daily. Consciousness never altered during or after attacks. He was then started on carbamazepine at dose of 100 mg twice daily, which resulted in complete resolution of his signs.

The neurological examination revealed negative signs of cranial nerves, normal muscle strength and tension, sensation, and deep tendon reflexes. The Babinski sign was bilaterally negative. Blood routine, blood smear, ferritin, and ceruloplasmin revealed no significant findings. EEG showed unremarkable findings. The brain MRI scanning was uninformative.

His father had similar attacks between 15 and 30 years old (Fig. 4.3). The involuntary movements usually occurred when initiating walking, running, or standing up. These episodes gradually disappeared after the age of 30. His mother and brother were asymptomatic. The physical examination was essentially normal in his father, mother, and brother.

Fig. 4.3 The pedigree chart of the family. *Squares* indicate males; *circles* demonstrate females; the *black symbols* depict affected individuals; *arrows* indicate the proband

Primary Diagnosis

This case mainly presented with repeated and paroxysmal choreoathetosis. His neurological examinations, laboratory tests, EEG, and brain MRI are essentially uninformative. According to his symptoms, the localization most likely involves extrapyramidal system or cerebral cortex. A positive history with autosomal dominant inheritance suggests that heredity may be the main etiology of his attacks. His periodic, transitory, and repeated episodes highly resemble the seizure attacks or transient ischemic attack (TIA). However, the fully preserved consciousness during the attacks suggests that epilepsy is less likely. His symmetrical spells and exciting symptoms imply the little possibility of TIA. The paroxysmal choreoathetosis with undisturbed consciousness hints a diagnosis of paroxysmal dyskinesias (PDs), which include paroxysmal kinesigenic dyskinesia (PKD), paroxysmal non-kinesigenic dyskinesia (PNKD), and paroxysmal exercise-induced dyskinesia (PED). The patient described here had a trigger of sudden movement, consistent with the features of PKD. Screening of *PRRT2* gene was necessary.

Additional Tests or Key Results

Sequencing of *PRRT2* gene was performed in this patient. We found heterozygous c.649dupC (p.R217Pfs*8) mutation in *PRRT2* (Fig. 4.4). Further investigations revealed that this mutation was also identified in his affected father but not in his asymptomatic mother and brother.

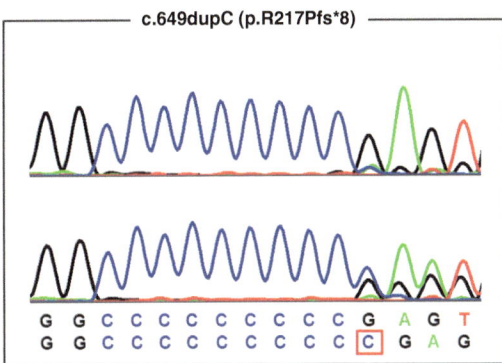

Fig. 4.4 Chromatogram of c.649dupC mutation in *PRRT2* gene. The *upper panel* depicts the normal sequence, while the *lower panel* indicates heterozygous mutated sequence

Discussion

PKD is a movement disorder with autosomal dominant inheritance and character of episodic involuntary movements which are usually triggered by sudden movement [10]. PKD attacks consist of chorea, athetosis, dystonia, and ballism, which are usually sudden, short, and relatively stereotyped. Consciousness is not altered during the attacks [11]. The frequency of episodes is variable among patients, ranging from 1 per month to 100 per day [12]. The symptoms usually commence in childhood or early adolescence and show a trend of remission with age in most cases. Stress and anxiety increase frequency of spells. It usually had favorable respond to antiepileptic drugs (AEDs), among which carbamazepine and phenytoin are priority drug. The causative gene of PKD is *PRRT2* which was located in 16p11.2

[13]. To date, more than 50 mutations within *PRRT2* have been reported, among which c.649dupC is a mutation hotspot worldwide [14].

This patient suffered from paroxysmal choreoathetosis which was usually triggered by sudden movement. The age at onset, precipitating factor, feature of attacks, and response to carbamazepine were all consistent with PKD. With the identification of *PRRT2* mutation, diagnosis of PKD is assured. PKD is the most common subtype of PDs. An important feature of PKD is the precipitating factor of sudden movement, which differentiates PKD from PNKD and PED. PNKD is usually triggered by substance like alcohol or coffee, menstruation, and strong emotion [15]. In contrast to PKD, PNKD attacks occur in lower frequency, last longer (10 min to 1 h), and respond poorly to AEDs [16]. The culprit gene of PNKD is *MR-1* [17]. PED is usually precipitated by prolonged exercise, and its attacks last several minutes (2–5 min on average) [18]. AEDs were usually not helpful for PED [19].

The good response to AEDs suggests that PKD may be an ion channel disease, although the underlying mechanisms remain largely unknown. Genotype–phenotype correlation of PKD revealed that patients carrying *PRRT2* mutations had earlier AAO and longer duration and tended to present with phenotype of dystonia and chorea [20, 21]. Among the AEDs, carbamazepine and phenytoin are the first selected drugs for patients with PKD. For the cases with *PRRT2* mutation, it was demonstrated that low-dose (50 mg/d) carbamazepine can completely resolve the attacks [20].

4.3   Dopa-Responsive Dystonia (DRD)

A 15-Year-Old Boy with Diurnal Fluctuation Abnormal Gait for 2 Years

Clinical Presentations

A 15-year-old boy came to our clinic with complaint of abnormal gait for 2 years. From the age of 13, he experienced a stiffness of right leg and gait disturbance. Two years later, he experienced stiffness and twisting in the trunk, the lower limbs, and right arm. All of the symptoms were improved in the morning, but aggravated toward the afternoon. He found it difficult to write and walk in the evening. The patient denied headaches, eyelid drooping, double vision, swallowing difficulty, or shortness of breath. His developmental history was unremarkable. He had no prior history of encephalitis, meningitis, febrile seizures, or head injury.

Neurologic examinations showed that cranial nerves were negative. His muscle strength was normal without muscle atrophy. The lower limbs muscular tension was increased. His lower limbs' deep tendon reflexes were exaggerated without ankle clonus. Hoffmann, Babinski, and Romberg signs were bilaterally negative. His deep and superficial sensation examinations were symmetric and normal. There were also no cerebellar impairment signs. The tiptoe gait was observed in the afternoon, but disappeared in the morning.

The blood routine examination was normal. Serum biochemistry analysis was normal (including lactic acid, uric acid, ceruloplasmin). The ophthalmic examinations excluded the presence of a Kayser–Fleisher (K–F) rings. The brain MRI disclosed unremarkable findings.

Interestingly, the patient's father, aged 40 years, developed similar symptoms at the age of 14 (Fig. 4.5a). The father manifested persistent posture tremor of upper extremities and torticollis around 20 years old. Whereas abnormal posture of his lower legs attenuated from his third decade. All the symptoms were mild after sleeping in the night, but aggravated in the afternoon and after exercise.

Primary Diagnosis

The patient showed muscle stiffness and twisting at the limbs and trunk; lower limbs' deep tendon reflexes were exaggerated without muscle weakness and Babinski signs. These symptoms were typically dystonia in which repetitive or sustained muscle contractions lead to twisting and repetitive movements or abnormal fixed postures. This disorder was presumed dysfunction of the basal ganglia.

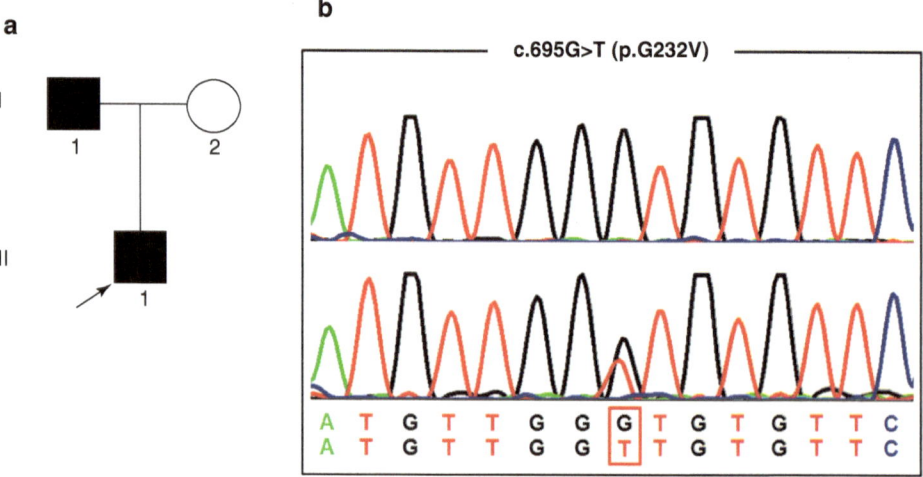

Fig. 4.5 Pedigree and mutation analysis of the patient. (**a**) The patient's pedigree chart. *Arrow* indicates the proband. (**b**) Chromatogram of p.G232V mutation within *GCH1* gene. The *upper panel* represents normal sequence of the control, whereas the *lower panel* is heterozygous mutated sequence of the patient

The disorder may be hereditary or caused by other factors such as birth related, infection, poisoning, or reaction to pharmaceutical drugs. The symptoms were childhood onset and positive family history, all of which implied that hereditary neurological disease should be considered first for this patient. The differential diagnosis includes dopa-responsive dystonia (DRD), Wilson's disease, juvenile-onset Parkinson's disease, and torsion dystonia. Wilson's disease was ruled out as the patient showed negative K–F ring and normal level of ceruloplasmin. Torsion dystonia was unlikely because the symptoms were diurnal fluctuation.

Subsequently, the trial of levodopa was propitious to differentiate dopa-responsive dystonia from other movement disorder. However, a positive response to levodopa does not differentiate DRD from juvenile-onset Parkinson's disease. Typically, patients with DRD will have a sustained benefit from low doses of levodopa without developing motor fluctuations and dyskinesia, in contrast to juvenile Parkinson's disease, in which these motor complications are a frequent occurrence. And most importantly, a gene test is necessary to confirm the diagnosis.

Additional Tests or Key Results

After treatment of 100 mg/day of levodopa for 3 days, the proband's symptoms were completely disappeared. He could walk and write normally in the evening. However, the father' posture tremor and torticollis were improved incompletely after administration of levodopa/benserazide (200 mg/day levodopa and 50 mg/day benserazide) for 10 days. The childhood onset of gait disturbance and dystonia mainly involved in lower limbs, noticeable diurnal fluctuation of those symptoms, a positive family history, and good response to levodopa strongly suggested the diagnosis of DRD. GCH1 gene analysis by direct sequencing of PCR product amplified was performed. Both of the proband and his father carried a heterozygous mutation c.695G>T in exon 6 of the GCH1 gene which would lead to a transition at codon 232 from a glycine to valine (Gly232Val) (Fig. 4.5b).

Discussion

DRD, also known as Segawa's disease, is a rare inherited disease with a prevalence of 1 per 2 million. This disorder is characterized by marked diurnal fluctuation, exquisite responsiveness to levodopa, and dystonia features. Clinical manifestations of DRD vary widely; patients with childhood onset may present with a posture dystonia, which typically starts in one leg. Some patients may show clubfoot and tiptoe walking due to the progression of dystonia. The symptoms can spread to other limbs in the early twenties, after which progression slows, and all symptoms reach a plateau at length. While adult-onset form may be action dystonia and parkinsonian feature, such signs may include torticollis, writing spasm, tremors, slowness of movement, stiffness, and balance difficulties. Approximately 25% of patients show abnormally exaggerated reflex responses in the legs [22, 23].

Both autosomal dominant and autosomal recessive forms of the DRD have been reported. The causative gene of autosomal dominant DRD is the GCH1 gene located on 14q22.1-q22.2 [24]. Mutation in the gene GCH1, which encodes the enzyme GTP cyclohydrolase I, disrupts the production of tetrahydrobiopterin (BH4). BH4 is the cofactor for dopamine synthesis. About 50–87% of DRD cases are caused by GCH1 mutations [25]. In the fewer autosomal recessive DRD, the mutations were reported in the genes for tyrosine hydroxylase and sepiapterin reductase. Tyrosine hydroxylase is the rate-limiting enzyme for dopamine synthesis. And sepiapterin reductase is also the cofactor for BH4 synthesis [26, 27].

In this DRD family, both of the patients have posture dystonia of lower legs in teens. However, the father exhibited posture tremor and torticollis several years later, which reflect that DRD patients have particular symptom in different age stage. The age-relative features are decided by dopa-relative pathway. It is the impairment of direct pathway and its descending output which mature early that lead to posture dystonia, while the involvement of subthalamic nucleus–internal segment and the globus pallidus–thalamus pathway that mature later causes tremor and torticollis, respectively [28]. However, these action dystonias were usually disabling and may be responsive to levodopa incompletely. These symptoms demanded further therapy, such as local injection of botulinum [29]. Therefore, early genetic diagnosis and therapy with small dose of levodopa for DRD patients in the age of adolescence may avoid developing into action dystonia later and bring patient long-term benefits.

4.4   Wilson's Disease (WD 1)

An 11-Year-Old Girl with Walking Difficulty and Slurred Speech

Clinical Presentations

An 11-year-old girl presented with walking difficulty for 10 months and slurred speech for 2 months. The girl was healthy at birth and grew up with normal developmental milestones. In the age of 10 years, the girl felt her legs were easier to get tired than usual after walking a long distance. At the same time, her parents noticed that her legs were gradually becoming misshapen with the emergence of knock-knees. Then the girl developed a knee pain while walking, which occurred more and more frequently and severely. The condition progressed so rapidly that the girl soon became unable to walk after 3 months. There were no symptoms of headache, tremors, or speech problems. Two months later, the girl underwent the orthopedic surgery for corrective therapy. However, 3 months after the surgery, she developed slurred speech, obvious drooling, slow swallowing, and writer's cramp. Her parents were worried about it and brought her to our clinic. There was no history of fever or loss of consciousness. She was not on any regular medications. Her parents and other family members did not have similar symptoms. Her parents said she had ever been hospitalized with liver dysfunction 5 years ago but had recovered and never recurred.

Neurological examinations revealed hypomimia and dysarthria. Her muscle force, tone, and reflexes were normal except an increased tone of upper limbs. Babinski sign was bilaterally negative. There were no signs of ataxia or sensory abnormalities. Routine blood count, liver and renal function, thyroid function, and serum electrolyte were normal. Notably, the abdominal ultrasonography showed a diffuse liver disease with nodules.

Primary Diagnosis

The history and examination revealed a bone deformity, liver disease, and neurological problems in childhood. The drooling, dysphagia, hypomimia, dysarthria, and increased tone in upper limbs suggested the impairments of extrapyramidal system. The differential diagnosis included Wilson's disease (WD), juvenile Parkinson's disease, early-onset primary dystonia, dopa-responsive dystonia (DRD), Niemann–Pick disease type C (NPC), drug effects or toxicity, central nervous system neoplasia, and hereditary ataxias. The multiple organ involvement implied the metabolic disorder like WD and NPC. However, the intact cerebellar function made the diagnosis of NPC highly unlikely. Brain imaging and biochemical tests were helpful to distinguish the WD with other non-metabolic diseases.

Additional Tests or Key Results

The serum ceruloplasmin was markedly decreased to level of 40 mg/L (reference, 200–400 mg/L), which highly suggested a diagnosis of WD. The serum copper was also lower (0.2 μg/mL) than normal (reference, 0.8–1.9 μg/mL). Her urinary copper of 24 h was elevated (484 μg, reference 0–100 μg). The ophthalmic examination confirmed the presence of Kayser–Fleisher (K–F) ring in her corneas (Fig. 4.6), which was sufficient to establish the diagnosis with the decreased ceruloplasmin. Consistently, magnetic resonance imaging (MRI) of the brain showed symmetrical T2-weighted hyperintense lesions in bilateral basal ganglia and thalami (Fig. 4.7). In addition, the *ATP7B* mutation analysis found compound heterozygous mutations, c.2621C>T (p.A874V) and c.2975C>T (p.P992L), which confirmed the diagnosis of WD (Fig. 4.8). The biallelic mutations were verified by the analysis of family members.

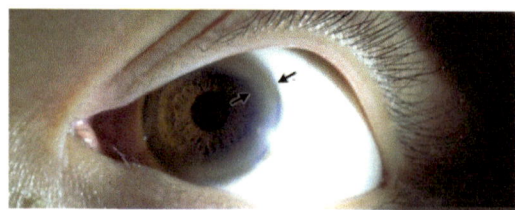

Fig. 4.6 The Kayser–Fleisher ring. Notice the green ring (*arrows*), which consists of copper deposits where the cornea meets the sclera

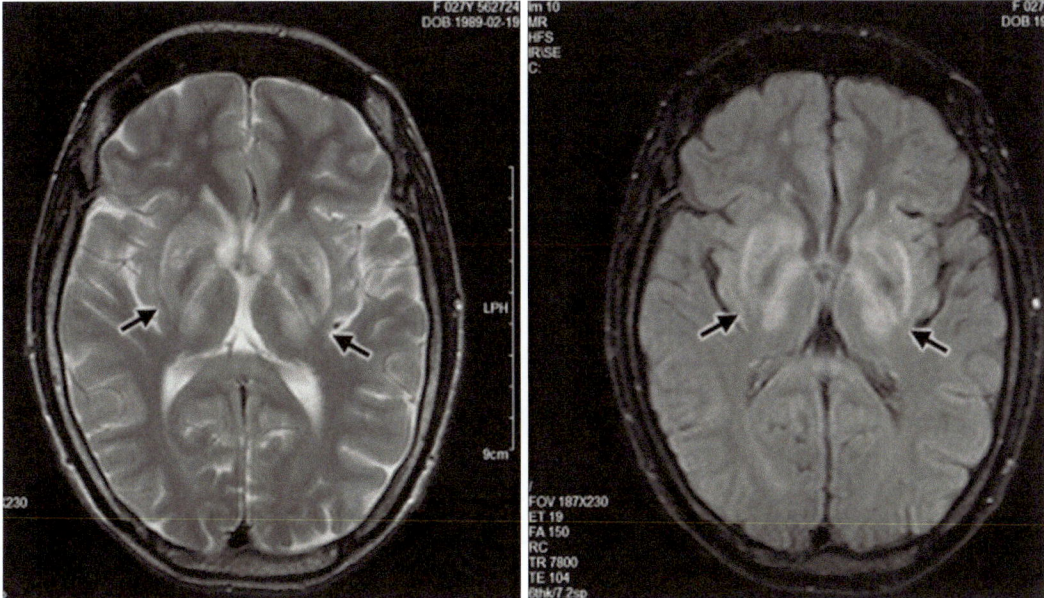

Fig. 4.7 Magnetic resonance imaging (MRI) of the brain in the patient. Axial MRI exhibits hyperintensity (*arrows*) in the bilateral lenticular nuclei and thalami on T2-weighted images (*left*) and T2-FLAIR (fluid-attenuated inversion recovery) images (*right*)

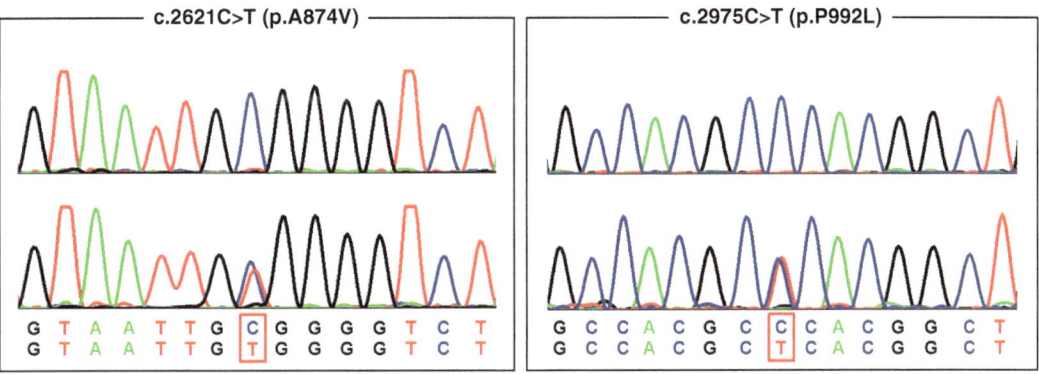

Fig. 4.8 Chromatogram of the *ATP7B* c.2621C>T (p.A874V) and c.2975C>T (p.P992L) mutations. The *upper panels* are normal sequences, whereas the *lower panels* represent mutated ones

Discussion

WD, also known as hepatolenticular degeneration, is an autosomal recessive disease (incidence 1/30,000) characterized by the color rings of corneas (K–F rings) and multisystem damage, including liver cirrhosis, extrapyramidal symptoms, psychiatric disorder, and musculoskeletal deformity. The disease is caused by mutations in ATP7B gene, which encodes a copper-transporting protein in the liver. A deficiency in the enzyme activity can lead to a toxic copper accumulation in multiple organs, which may be responsible for its wide variety of symptoms [30].

Despite a wide variety of clinical manifestations, WD typically presents with liver dysfunction or neurological disorders. Musculoskeletal abnormalities, including premature osteoarthritis, skeletal deformity, and pathological bone fractures, can be occasionally found in WD patients with hepatic or neurologic types [31, 32], but very rare as chief complains [33]. These conditions often lack typical hepatic and neurological symptoms, and the diagnosis can be challenging [34]. Most patients are never considered WD until the neurological impairments emerge, as in our patient. However, some typical signs of WD were present in our patient, such as K–F rings or abnormal abdominal ultrasonography.

In addition, the serum ceruloplasmin is a very sensitive test in WD patients even without any apparent hepatic and neurological signs. Ceruloplasmin below 0.1 g/L is highly suggestive of WD, but lower levels can also occur with aceruloplasminemia, malabsorption, renal or enteric protein loss, liver disease, and heterozygotes for WD [35]. Therefore, if the patient has a low-serum ceruloplasmin without K–F rings, the diagnosis should be based on combination of the urinary copper excretion, liver biopsy, and genetic test. Urinary copper excretion above 100 µg/24 h is

typical in patients with symptomatic WD, but less sensitive than ceruloplasmin and can be false positive with hepatic and renal disease. Liver biopsy is an invasive procedure and has been gradually substituted by genetic test. Genetic testing is confirmatory and convenient for screening family members.

The main treatment of WD is copper-chelating agents including D-penicillamine, trientine, dimercaptopropane sulfonate and dimercaptosuccinic acid, and zinc salts. Our patient took oral D-penicillamine (62.5 mg t.i.d.) combined with zinc gluconate (280 mg t.i.d.). After 1 year of follow-up, her symptoms of drooling, dysphagia, and writer's cramp relieved much.

In summary, when a child or adolescent presents with unexplained joint pain or bone dysplasia, the possibility of WD should be considered. Biochemical tests, abdominal ultrasound, slit-light examination, and brain MRI can help establish the diagnosis. Earlier diagnosis can initiate an earlier treatment and prevent the further damage.

4.5   Wilson's Disease (WD 2)

A 22-Year-Old Male Presented with Abnormal Behavior for 10 Months

Clinical Presentations

A Chinese male patient, aged 22, was referred to the Clinic of Neurology due to abrupt behavior change. According to his comrades, the affected individual was noted to soliloquize and have insomnia over the past 10 months. Sometimes he behaved weirdly in front of his comrades and became to be easily irritated with increased hostility toward comrades. There is no family history of any mental disorders. His birth, developmental milestones, and early childhood are normal.

On admission, complete physical examinations revealed practically normal somatic signs, including afebrile, eupneic breathing, normal heart rate, and normotensive without the occurrence of organomegaly. On mental state examination, he was easily irritable and provocative. He has poor control of aggressive personality, hypersensitivity, and soliloquy. Neurological examinations, including extrapyramidal system, all showed normal.

During the primary evaluation, his routine tests in the form of hemogram, renal function, and brain magnetic resonance imaging (MRI) did not display any abnormality. However, liver function (ALT, 46 U/L; normal range is 8–40 U/L) and ultrasound examination of the abdomen revealed moderate impairment.

Primary Diagnosis

Based on his clinical presentations, diagnosis of schizophrenia was initially made for him by psychiatrists from two different hospitals. Therefore, he began to take antipsychotic medications including risperidone and benzhexol. However, after receiving regular therapy, his distress did not improve significantly.

After 10 months, he was presented to a general practitioner who subsequently referred him to genetic clinic. We carefully reviewed his disease course and the related test results. Moderate liver function abnormalities were observed during the overall disease course, even before receiving medication treatment.

Additional Tests or Key Results

In addition, when we evaluated Kayser–Fleischer (K–F) rings using a slit lamp, noted K–F rings were found in his eyes. Therefore, other laboratory tests, including 24-h urinary copper excretion and ceruloplasmin level, were further carried out in the affected individual. Consequently, the low-serum ceruloplasmin level (0.03 g/L, reference value is 0.15–0.31 g/L) was observed, whereas urinary copper was normal. Therefore, this case was highly suggestive of Wilson's disease (WD) and screened for *ATP7B*, which is causative gene of WD patient. Genetic test demonstrated that the patient harbored two heterogeneous mutations, including p.R778L and p.V1106I (Fig. 4.9), thus confirming the diagnosis of WD.

Discussion

WD is an inherited disorder of copper metabolism due to ATP7B protein dysfunction, which mainly affects the liver and central nervous system. Clinical profile often includes hepatic, neurologic, or psychiatric disturbance or a combination of these [30]. Liver disease may be in the form of recurrent jaundice, elevated transaminase level, and chronic liver disease or cirrhosis, while neurological manifestations may include choreiform movements, rigidity, gait disturbance, tremors, dysarthria, etc.

The psychiatric findings are variable and can span a range of diagnostic entities. Depression, cognitive impairment, and personality changes are the most common findings in WD patients with psychiatric form [36]. Compared to these presentations, schizophreniform symptoms are less commonly observed in patients with WD. A clinical investigation from India revealed that only three cases presented with schizophreniform among 350 affected individuals [37]. Grover et al. reported that the overall prevalence of psychosis in patients with WD varies from 0 to 11.3% [38]. Although psychiatric disturbances are well known in WD, the exclusive psychiatric

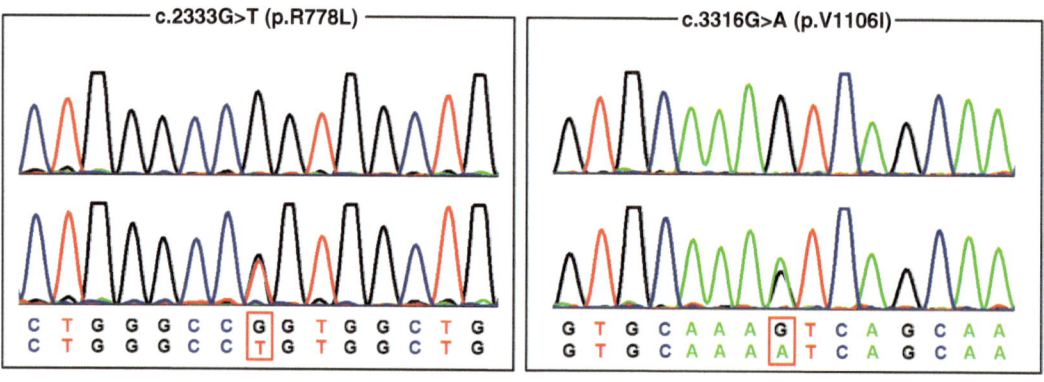

Fig. 4.9 Chromatogram of the *ATPTB* p.R778L and p.V1106I mutations. The *upper panel* represents normal sequence, while the *lower panel* being heterozygous mutated sequence

manifestation mimicking a schizophrenic psychosis without noted hepatic or neurological disorders is relatively rare.

In our case study, the affected individual initially presented with psychosis disturbances and was given the wrong treatment as a schizophrenic patient. Combined with other reports, early recognitions to WD patients only with psychiatric abnormalities are critical because timely initiation of chelation therapy can prevent a catastrophic outcome. We feel that WD diagnostic possibility should be suspected in patients experiencing with abrupt neuropsychiatric symptoms, especially accompanied by unknown liver function abnormalities and abdominal ultrasound for architectural alternation in liver.

4.6 Pantothenate Kinase-Associated Neurodegeneration (PKAN)

A 47-Year-Old Man Had Involuntary Movement for 1 Year

Clinical Presentations

A 47-year-old male came to our Department of Neurology because of involuntary movement for 1 year. He is a shopkeeper and denied any history of toxic exposure. Without any precipitating factor, he suffered from intermittent hypsokinesis of head last year. The attacks usually last 1–3 s and occurred 3–5 times per day. It was mainly involved in his head and occasionally in his neck. There were no convulsions, tremor of limbs, or consciousness alteration during the episodes. He was diagnosed with physiological tremor in local hospital and was prescribed arotinolol hydrochloride at dose of 5 mg thrice daily, which did not relieve his symptoms at all. Four months later, he found his symptoms were aggravated, as the frequency was increased to 5–10 times per day. When he sought his medical attentions in our hospital, he presented apparent dystonic posturing of head. His older brother and parents were all asymptomatic. He denied any family history of consanguinity or neurological disorders.

Cranial nerves examination revealed negative signs except for the involuntary movement of head. The muscle strength was 5/5 in four limbs, and muscle tension was essentially normal. There was no abnormality of somatosensory. Deep reflex was symmetrical and pathological sign was bilaterally negative. Ataxia was not observed. His recognition was not impaired, with MMSE score of 29/30. Complete blood count, T3 T4, ceruloplasmin, serum ferritin, albumin, and lipoproteins were in normal range. Brain MRI showed bilateral hyperintensity within surrounding hypointensity in the globus pallidus on T2 weighted (Fig. 4.10a) and T2-FLAIR (Fig. 4.10b). Susceptibility-weighted image (SWI) revealed low hypointensity in the globus pallidus (Fig. 4.10c).

Primary Diagnosis

This patient mainly presented repeated and intermittent hypsokinesis of head, which resembles the feature of dystonia. There was no sign of pyramidal tracts and cerebellum in physical examination. The level diagnosis was thus located in extrapyramidal tract. Adult onset, slow progression, and no relapsing-remitting episode excluded the infection, inflammation, vessel, and trauma as the etiologic diagnosis of disease. Metabolism, intoxication, degeneration, and heredity should be considered. Showed as in SWI

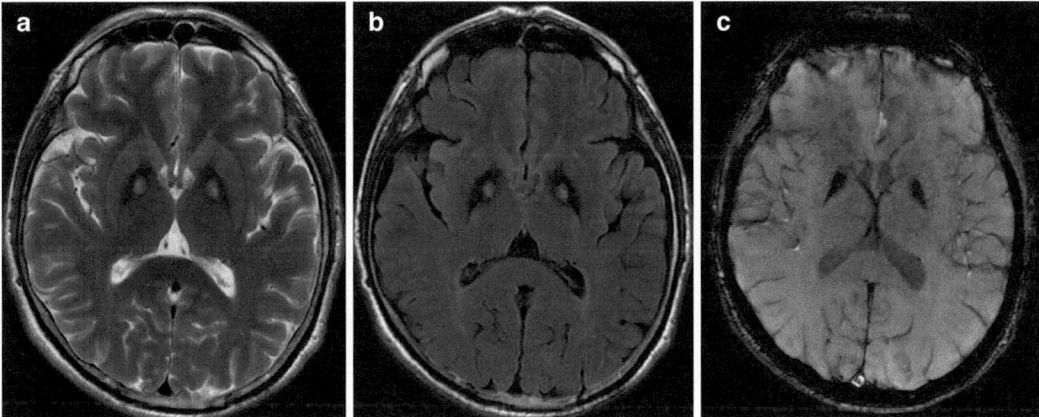

Fig. 4.10 Brain MRI of the patient revealed bilateral hyperintensity within surrounding hypointensity in the globus pallidus on T2 weighted (**a**) and T2-FLAIR (**b**). Susceptibility-weighted image (SWI) revealed low hypointensity in the globus pallidus (**c**)

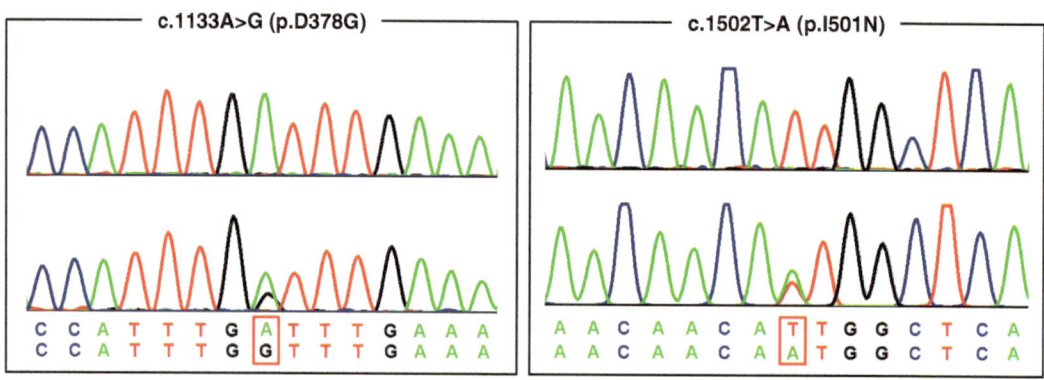

Fig. 4.11 Chromatogram of c.1133A>G (p.D378G) and c.1502 T>A (p.I501N) in *PANK2* gene. The *upper panel* indicates the normal sequence, and the *lower panel* shows heterozygous mutation

sequence, the low hypointensity in the globus pallidus implied the deposition of iron. Extrapyramidal symptoms and iron accumulation in globus pallidus implied that neurodegeneration with brain iron accumulation (NBIA) was the paramount consideration.

Additional Tests or Key Results

There are ten subtypes of NBIA and the majority is autosomal recessive inherited [39]. Among the NBIA groups, pantothenate kinase-associated neurodegeneration (PKAN) is the most common type, accounting for 30–50% NBIA cases. Therefore, genetic screening of *PANK2* gene should be first conducted. After sequencing of *PANK2* gene, we identified two heterozygous c.1133A>G (p. D378G) and c.1502 T>A (p.I501N) mutations in the proband (Fig. 4.11). Further investigation demonstrated that his father carried c.1502 T>A mutation and his mother carried c.1133A>G mutation.

Discussion

PKAN is a rare neurodegenerative disorder with autosomal recessive inheritance and iron accumulation in the globus pallidus [40]. Previously, this disorder was well-known as Hallervorden–Spatz syndrome and renamed in 2011. Clinically, PKAN is characterized by early onset of extrapyramidal symptoms and rapid progression [41]. Nevertheless, a fraction of cases with atypical PKAN had relatively late AAO and slower progression [42, 43]. Due to the recessive inheritance,

family history is usually inconspicuous, resulting in the missed diagnosis of this disorder. "Eye-of-the-tiger" sign is a specific imaging feature in PKAN. It was shown as symmetrical hypointensity with a central region of hyperintensity in globus pallidus.

This patient presented with neck dystonia at age of 46. We did not consider hereditary diseases at first because of his onset of adulthood, 1-year disease course, and negative family history. However, his brain MRI revealed classic "eye-of-the-tiger" sign, which is a crucial clue for the diagnosis of PKAN. "Eye-of-the-tiger" sign is a specific imaging feature. It is mainly seen in PKAN and occasionally observed in neuroacanthocytosis and other conditions. In this case, we also performed peripheral blood smear but did not find increased number of acanthocytes (>5%). Neuroacanthocytosis was therefore excluded. He was detected to carry compound heterozygous PANK2 mutations, which co-segregated with the disease. He was finally diagnosed with PKAN.

Current treatment in PKAN is primarily symptomatic for relief of spasticity, dystonia, and other movement disorder. Commonly used drugs are benzodiazepines, anticholinergic, baclofen, neuroleptics, and L-dopa. Deep brain stimulation (DBS) causes mild improvement in dystonia severity [44], and no definite result has been achieved by iron-chelating agents (such as deferiprone) in clinical trials [45].

4.7   Neuroacanthocytosis

A 41-Year-Old Man with Unsteadiness and Memory Impairment

Clinical Presentations

A 41-year-old male presented to us with a 4-year history of increasing unsteady on his feet. At first, he noticed "heaviness" in his legs, particularly while climbing up stairs. Sometimes, he felt his knees bent forward involuntary while walking. These symptoms were subtle at the beginning and progressed gradually. His wife reported that he had difficulties in concentrating and felt that he was increasingly forgetful for the latest 2 years, and he lost his job due to the memory impairment. He reported no sensory symptoms and no symptoms of bladder or bowel dysfunction. He was admitted to our Neurology Department for further examinations. He has been systemically well with no weight loss, change in appetite, or sleep habit. He takes no alcohol or cigarette or regular medications. On examinations, the general systemic examinations including blood pressure was unremarkable. His Mini-Mental State Examination (MMSE) score was 29/30 dropping only 1 point for attention and calculation. His cranial nerves were entirely normal. The limbs were normal on inspection, with no wasting or fasciculations. Tone was normal; power was symmetrically normal 5/5 in all muscle groups in the legs and throughout the arms. All reflexes were decreased and plantars were mute. The coordination was generally good with slight clumsy of hands rotation.

The blood tests were all grossly normal apart from a creatine kinase (CK) of 2244 U/L (reference < 171 U/L) and CK-MB 50 U/L (reference < 24 U/L). His ECG and echocardiogram were normal. Electromyography (EMG) showed widespread slowing of conduction in sensory and motor nerves (Table 4.1). An MRI scan of the brain demonstrated slight cortical atrophy.

The electromyography findings showed that the motor conduction velocities of common peroneus were slow, and motor-induced amplitudes were reduced. The sensory conduction velocities of sural were slow, and sensory-induced amplitudes were also slightly decreased.

Primary Diagnosis

The history and examination findings suggest that this patient has a diffuse impairment of the nervous system including peripheral nerves, muscles, and possibly cortical function. This is far more likely to be a certain complex syndrome. Because the most severe impairment was the elevated CK level, we considered myopathy to be the first diagnosis, of which mitochondrial encephlomyopathyis of great possibility. Further questioning revealed that he was not good at sports since a child, and his unsteadiness always developed when he felt tired. Although the decrease in exercise tolerance may simply represent fatigue, in this case it may highly signify neurological muscle weakness affecting the limbs that argue strongly in favor of a possible diagnosis of mitochondrial encephalomyopathy. We tested the serum lactic acid level after

Table 4.1 Nerve conduction study

Nerve	Stimulate point	Latency (ms)	Amplitude (mV)	Velocity (m/s)
Motor nerve conduction velocity (MCV)				
Peroneus (L)	Ankle	6.25	1.51	
	Capitula fibula	14.1	0.94	34.3
Peroneus (R)	Ankle	3.76	4.0	
	Capitula fibula	10.5	3.5	40.9
Sensory nerve conduction velocity (SCV)				
Sural (L)	14 cm above heel	2.18	7.1	39.0
Sural (R)	14 cm above heel	2.07	5.0	36.2

exercise. The lactic acid levels were 1.6 mmol/L at rest, 5.2 mmol/L immediately after exercise, 4.6 mmol/L 10 min after exercise, and 2.2 mmol/L 30 min after exercise, while the reference range is 0.7–2.1 mmol/L. Although these results meet the minimum diagnosis criteria for mitochondria disease, the lactic level is often much higher. Muscle biopsy is considered to perform in the patient.

Additional Tests or Key Results

Before muscle biopsy was scheduled, on further physical examinations, we noticed that there were some involuntary fidgeting, writhing, and twitching movements of the distal of limbs. The movements appear semi-purposeful but in a random pattern. They were very subtle thus could only be noticed on a long time careful observation. These involuntary movements were chore form, thus reminding us the possibility of Huntington's disease (HD). However, the increased CK level and peripheral neuropathy could not be explained by HD. HD genotyping was requested and negative, which excluded the diagnosis of HD. The complex presentations that include peripheral neuropathy, cortical function impairment, chore form involuntary movements, as well as an increased CK level raise the suspicion of a rare inherited disorder, neuroacanthocytosis (NA). Peripheral blood smear was performed, and an increased number of acanthocytes (>5%) were found (Fig. 4.12) and supported the diagnosis of NA. A detailed family history reveals that no one in his family experienced similar symptoms reminding us the possibility of an X-linked recessive inheritance. McLeod syndrome (MLS) is one of NA syndromes and an X-linked recessive disorder caused by mutations of *XK* gene located on the X chromosome [46]. Therefore, mutations of *XK* were screened in the patient, and the c.942G>A (p.W314X) mutation was found (Fig. 4.13), which further confirmed the diagnosis of MLS.

Discussion

NA is a group of very rare disorders estimated to have affected 1000 people worldwide. There are four core NA syndromes including chorea-acanthocytosis (ChAc), MLS, Huntington's disease-like 2 (HDL2), and pantothenate kinase-

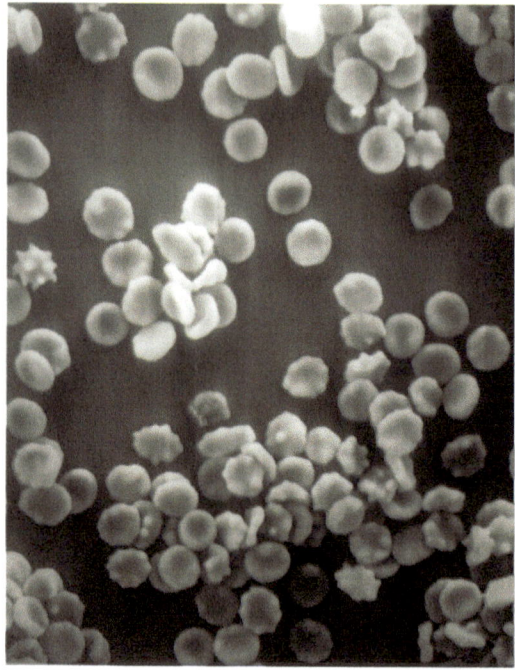

Fig. 4.12 Peripheral blood smear on electron microscope showed an increased number of acanthocytes (>5%)

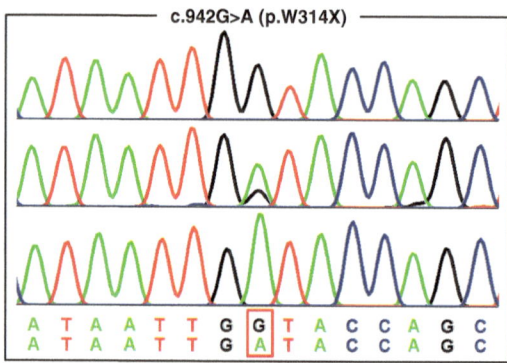

Fig. 4.13 Mutation analysis of the patient. Chromatogram of c.942G>A (p.W314X) mutation in *XK* gene. The *upper panel* is normal sequence of the control, the *middle panel* represents the heterozygous c.942G>A sequence, whereas the *lower panel* represents hemizygous c.942G>A sequence of the patient

associated neurodegeneration (PKAN) [47]. MLS typically presents in men in their midlife with hyperkinetic involuntary movements, specifically chorea, peripheral sensorimotor neuropathy, psychiatric or cognitive issues, and an elevated CK or liver enzymes. Fifty percent of subjects have seizures, which usually respond well to standard anticonvulsant medications. The main observation on brain imaging is atrophy of the caudate nucleus and putamen [48].

Our diagnosis of MLS was first based on clinical features and laboratory findings. Clinically, the patient had midlife onset illness. Hence, our diagnosis was restricted to either ChAc or MLS because HDL2 and PKAN have a childhood or juvenile onset. However, because the characteristic phenotype of ChAc including a very peculiar "feeding dystonia" with tongue protrusion, orofacial dyskinesias, and involuntary tongue/lip biting was absent in our patient, our first diagnosis was MLS. In addition, an important distinction between MLS and the other NA disorders is the presence of cardiomyopathy [49], which is seen in approximately 2/3 of patients. Although the ECG and echocardiogram of this patient were normal, he did have an increased CK-MB level (50 U/L, reference <24 U/L).

The diagnosis of this patient was quite difficult at beginning because his chore form movement was too subtle to be recognized. However, on retrospection, the combination of symptoms should raise our suspicion of NA even without the hyperkinetic involuntary movements. In conclusion, although NA disorders are rare, the clinical presentations are very characteristic that should be recognized [50].

References

1. Dorsey ER, Constantinescu R, Thompson JP, Biglan KM, Holloway RG, Kieburtz K, et al. Projected number of people with Parkinson disease in the most populous nations, 2005 through 2030. Neurology. 2007;68(5):384–6.
2. Lees AJ, Hardy J, Revesz T. Parkinson's disease. Lancet. 2009;373(9680):2055–66.
3. Bonifati V. Autosomal recessive parkinsonism. Parkinsonism Relat Disord. 2012;18(Suppl 1):S4–6.
4. Sun M, Latourelle JC, Wooten GF, Lew MF, Klein C, Shill HA, et al. Influence of heterozygosity for parkin mutation on onset age in familial Parkinson disease: the GenePD study. Arch Neurol. 2006;63(6):826–32.
5. Deng H, Le W, Shahed J, Xie W, Jankovic J. Mutation analysis of the parkin and PINK1 genes in American Caucasian early-onset Parkinson disease families. Neurosci Lett. 2008;430(1):18–22.
6. Khan NL, Horta W, Eunson L, Graham E, Johnson JO, Chang S, et al. Parkin disease in a Brazilian kindred: manifesting heterozygotes and clinical follow-up over 10 years. Mov Disord. 2005;20(4):479–84.
7. Khan NL, Graham E, Critchley P, Schrag AE, Wood NW, Lees AJ, et al. Parkin disease: a phenotypic study of a large case series. Brain. 2003;126(Pt 6):1279–92.
8. Lohmann E, Periquet M, Bonifati V, Wood NW, De Michele G, Bonnet AM, et al. How much phenotypic variation can be attributed to parkin genotype? Ann Neurol. 2003;54(2):176–85.
9. Pahwa R, Lyons KE. Treatment of early Parkinson's disease. Curr Opin Neurol. 2014;27(4):442–9.
10. Ream M, Morgan-Followell B, Ghosh D. Paroxysmal kinesigenic dyskinesia: seeing is believing. Pediatr Neurol. 2015;53(4):369–70.
11. Youn J, Kim JS, Lee M, Lee J, Roh H, Ki CS, et al. Clinical manifestations in paroxysmal kinesigenic dyskinesia patients with proline-rich transmembrane protein 2 gene mutation. J Clin Neurol. 2014;10(1):50–4.
12. Demirkiran M, Jankovic J. Paroxysmal dyskinesias: clinical features and classification. Ann Neurol. 1995;38(4):571–9.
13. Chen WJ, Lin Y, Xiong ZQ, Wei W, Ni W, Tan GH, et al. Exome sequencing identifies truncating mutations in PRRT2 that cause paroxysmal kinesigenic dyskinesia. Nat Genet. 2011;43(12):1252–5.
14. Heron SE, Dibbens LM. Role of PRRT2 in common paroxysmal neurological disorders: a gene with remarkable pleiotropy. J Med Genet. 2013;50(3):133–9.
15. Peila E, Mortara P, Cicerale A, Pinessi L. Paroxysmal non-kinesigenic dyskinesia, post-streptococcal syndromes and psychogenic movement disorders: a diagnostic challenge. BMJ Case Rep. 2015;2015: bcr2014207449.
16. Bruno MK, Lee HY, Auburger GW, Friedman A, Nielsen JE, Lang AE, et al. Genotype-phenotype correlation of paroxysmal nonkinesigenic dyskinesia. Neurology. 2007;68(21):1782–9.
17. Rainier S, Thomas D, Tokarz D, Ming L, Bui M, Plein E, et al. Myofibrillogenesis regulator 1 gene mutations cause paroxysmal dystonic choreoathetosis. Arch Neurol. 2004;61(7):1025–9.
18. Tacik P, Loens S, Schrader C, Gayde-Stephan S, Biskup S, Dressler D. Severe familial paroxysmal exercise-induced dyskinesia. J Neurol. 2014;261(10): 2009–15.
19. Bhatia KP. Paroxysmal dyskinesias. Mov Disord. 2011;26(6):1157–65.
20. Li HF, Chen WJ, Ni W, Wang KY, Liu GL, Wang N, et al. PRRT2 mutation correlated with phenotype of paroxysmal kinesigenic dyskinesia and drug response. Neurology. 2013;80(16):1534–5.
21. Huang XJ, Wang T, Wang JL, Liu XL, Che XQ, Li J, et al. Paroxysmal kinesigenic dyskinesia: clinical and genetic analyses of 110 patients. Neurology. 2015; 85(18):1546–53.
22. Segawa M. Hereditary progressive dystonia with marked diurnal fluctuation. Brain Dev. 2011;33(3): 195–201.

23. Wijemanne S, Jankovic J. Dopa-responsive dystonia—clinical and genetic heterogeneity. Nat Rev Neurol. 2015;11(7):414–24.

24. Rose SJ, Yu XY, Heinzer AK, Harrast P, Fan X, Raike RS, Thompson VB, Pare JF, Weinshenker D, Smith Y, Jinnah HA, Hess EJ. A new knock-in mouse model of l-DOPA-responsive dystonia. Brain. 2015;138(Pt 10):2987–3002.

25. Wu ZY, Lin Y, Chen WJ, Zhao GX, Xie H, Murong SX, Wang N. Molecular analyses of GCH-1, TH and parkin genes in Chinese dopa-responsive dystonia families. Clin Genet. 2008;74(6):513–21.

26. Abeling NG, Duran M, Bakker HD, Stroomer L, Thony B, Blau N, Booij J, Poll-The BT. Sepiapterin reductase deficiency an autosomal recessive DOPA-responsive dystonia. Mol Genet Metab. 2006; 89(1–2):116–20.

27. Steinberger D, Blau N, Goriuonov D, Bitsch J, Zuker M, Hummel S, Muller U. Heterozygous mutation in 5′-untranslated region of sepiapterin reductase gene (SPR) in a patient with dopa-responsive dystonia. Neurogenetics. 2004;5(3):187–90.

28. Lin Y, Wang DN, Chen WJ, Lin X, Lin MT, Wang N. Growth hormone deficiency in a dopa-responsive dystonia patient with a novel mutation of guanosine triphosphate cyclohydrolase 1 gene. J Child Neurol. 2015;30(6):796–9.

29. van den Dool J, Tijssen MA, Koelman JH, Engelbert RH, Visser B. Determinants of disability in cervical dystonia. Parkinsonism Relat Disord. 2016;32:48–53.

30. Huster D. Wilson disease. Best Pract Res Clin Gastroenterol. 2010;24(5):531–9.

31. Balint G, Szebenyi B. Hereditary disorders mimicking and/or causing premature osteoarthritis. Baillieres Best Pract Res Clin Rheumatol. 2000;14(2):219–50.

32. Quemeneur AS, Trocello JM, Ea HK, Woimant F, Liote F. Miscellaneous non-inflammatory musculoskeletal conditions. Musculoskeletal conditions associated with Wilson's disease. Best Pract Res Clin Rheumatol. 2011;25(5):627–36.

33. Cai YZ, Jiang TZ, Yang RM. Osseomuscular type of hepatolenticular degeneration: report of 11 cases. Lin Chuang Shen Jing Bing Xue Za Zhi. 1994;7(3):142–4.

34. Dastur DK, Manghani DK, Wadia NH. Wilson's disease in India. I. Geographic, genetic, and clinical aspects in 16 families. Neurology. 1968;18(1 Pt 1):21–31.

35. European Association for Study of Liver. EASL clinical practice guidelines: Wilson's disease. J Hepatol. 2012;56(3):671–85.

36. Wichowicz HM, Cubala WJ, Slawek J. Wilson's disease associated with delusional disorder. Psychiatry Clin Neurosci. 2006;60(6):758–60.

37. Srinivas K, Sinha S, Taly AB, Prashanth LK, Arunodaya GR, Janardhana Reddy YC, et al. Dominant psychiatric manifestations in Wilson's disease: a diagnostic and therapeutic challenge! J Neurol Sci. 2008;266(1–2):104–8.

38. Grover S, Sarkar S, Jhanda S, Chawla Y. Psychosis in an adolescent with Wilson's disease: a case report and review of the literature. Indian J Psychiatry. 2014; 56(4):395–8.

39. Schneider SA. Neurodegeneration with brain iron accumulation. Curr Neurol Neurosci Rep. 2016; 16(1):9.

40. Ma LY, Wang L, Yang YM, Lu Y, Cheng FB, Wan XH. Novel gene mutations and clinical features in patients with pantothenate kinase-associated neurodegeneration. Clin Genet. 2015;87(1):93–5.

41. Hayflick SJ, Westaway SK, Levinson B, Zhou B, Johnson MA, Ching KH, et al. Genetic, clinical, and radiographic delineation of Hallervorden-Spatz syndrome. N Engl J Med. 2003;348(1):33–40.

42. Lee JH, Park J, Ryu HS, Park H, Kim YE, Hong JY, et al. Clinical heterogeneity of atypical pantothenate kinase-associated neurodegeneration in Koreans. J Mov Disord. 2016;9(1):20–7.

43. Tomic A, Petrovic I, Svetel M, Dobricic V, Dragasevic Miskovic N, Kostic VS. Pattern of disease progression in atypical form of pantothenate-kinase-associated neurodegeneration (PKAN): prospective study. Parkinsonism Relat Disord. 2015; 21(5):521–4.

44. Sathe KP, Hegde AU, Doshi PK. Deep brain stimulation improves quality of life in pantothenate kinase-associated neurodegeneration. J Pediatr Neurosci. 2013;8(1):46–8.

45. Pratini NR, Sweeters N, Vichinsky E, Neufeld JA. Treatment of classic pantothenate kinase-associated neurodegeneration with deferiprone and intrathecal baclofen. Am J Phys Med Rehabil. 2013;92(8): 728–33.

46. Ho M, Chelly J, Carter N, Danek A, Crocker P, Monaco AP. Isolation of the gene for McLeod syndrome that encodes a novel membrane transport protein. Cell. 1994;77(6):869–80.

47. Walker RH. Untangling the thorns: advances in the neuroacanthocytosis syndromes. J Mov Disord. 2015;8(2):41–54.

48. Valko PO, Hanggi J, Meyer M, Jung HH. Evolution of striatal degeneration in McLeod syndrome. Eur J Neurol. 2010;17(4):612–8.

49. Oechslin E, Kaup D, Jenni R, Jung HH. Cardiac abnormalities in McLeod syndrome. Int J Cardiol. 2009;132(1):130–2.

50. Walker RH. Management of neuroacanthocytosis syndromes. Tremor Other Hyperkinet Mov. 2015;5:346.

Yu Lin

Abstract

Ion channel diseases are diseases caused by dysfunction of ion channel subunits or the regular proteins. Ion channels are essential in neuronal signaling and thus channelopathies can be found in skeletal muscle or central nervous system diseases, which include hyperkalemic and hypokalemic periodic paralysis, episodic ataxia, familial hemiplegic migraine, generalized epilepsy with febrile seizures plus and so on. These diseases can be either acquired or inherited. Since 1990, many mutations in genes encoding ion channel components have been discovered to cause disorders. The findings of genetic causes contribute to explain similarities and differences in clinical and laboratory manifestations in these disorders. In this chapter, we presented two commonly encountered ion channel diseases caused by genetic mutations.

Keywords

Ion channel diseases • Hyperkalemic periodic paralysis • Hypokalemic periodic paralysis

Y. Lin
Department of Neurology, First Affiliated Hospital,
Fujian Medical University, Fuzhou, China
e-mail: yulinwin2009@aliyun.com

5.1 Hypokalemic Periodic Paralysis

The 29-Year-Old Woman with Recurrent Weakness of the Extremities

Clinical Presentations

The 29-year-old woman admitted to our hospital complained of recurrent weakness of the extremities. She had experienced the first attack of paralysis for several hours in all extremities upon waking since 4 years old. The symptoms occurred during awakening or after sleep or rest following strenuous exercise. The frequency of attacks was less than 20 times per year. The patient denied any weight loss, anxiety, palpitations, tremors, diarrhea, or increased perspiration. She was not on any medications and denied smoking, alcohol, or illicit drug abuse. Family history showed that her son also had a history of periodic paralysis since he was 2 years old, but the severity and frequency of the attacks relieved at the age of 4 (Fig. 5.1a).

Neurological examination revealed proximal limbs weakness with a symmetrical power score of 1/5 in the lower extremities and 3/5 in the upper extremities. Sensory and cerebellar were normal. Deep tendon reflexes were diminished. The rest of the physical examination was unremarkable.

Laboratory data revealed a low serum potassium level of 1.8 mmol/L (reference range 3.5–5.4). Routine blood parameters including serum creatine kinase level were normal. Thyroid function tests were normal. The ECG examination revealed sinus rhythm with flattened T waves and notably U waves.

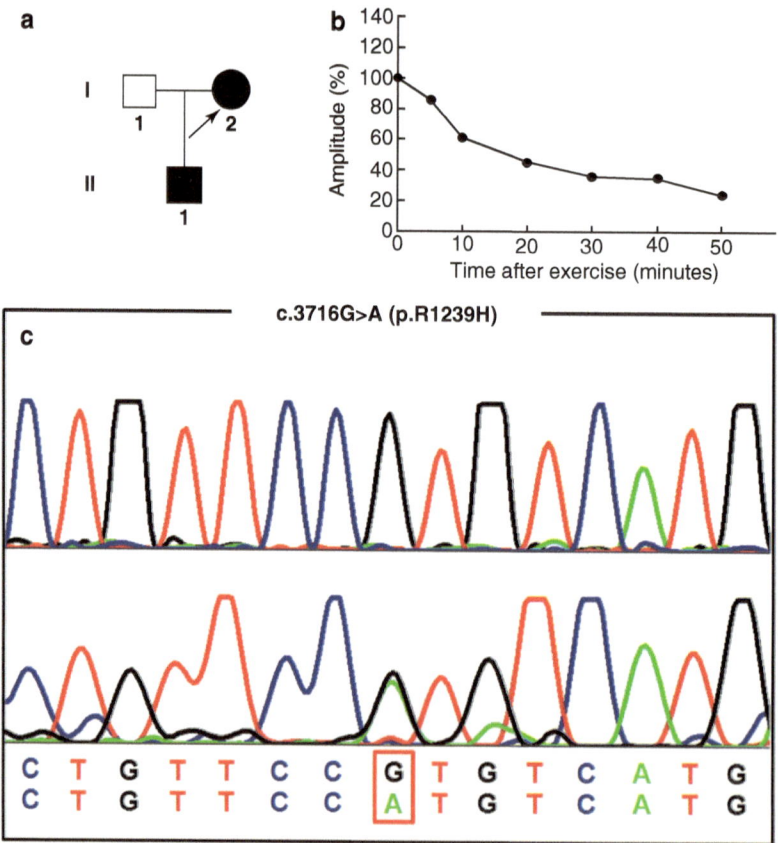

Fig. 5.1 (a) The patient's pedigree chart. *Arrow* indicates the proband. (b) Long exercise test showed amplitudes of CMAPs denoted as a percentage of its pre-exercise value are plotted against the time elapsed after 5 min of exercise. The results of CMAP amplitudes are noted as a percentage, where the 100% mean CMAP amplitudes obtained during the pre-excise period. (c) Sequencing chromatograms showing the heterozygous p.R1239H mutant in *CACNA1S* gene. In the mutant sequence, the G-to-A transition at CDNA position 3716 results in the replacement of Arg by His at codon 1239

Primary Diagnosis

The clinical manifestation is episodic weakness associated with low serum potassium levels. The attack was triggered in resting state following strenuous exercise. Neurological examination revealed weakness of proximal muscle. Sensory and cerebellar were normal. Tendon reflexes of limbs were diminished. These signs hinted that the paralysis was due to lesions of the lower motor neurons. Because the sensory disturbance was absent, the lesion must be situated in a motor branch of a peripheral nerve, in motor neurons alone, in the neuromuscular junction, or in the muscle itself. The differential diagnosis of a young female with episodes of flaccid weakness included periodic paralysis, myasthenia gravis, and Lambert-Eaton syndromes.

Subsequently, EMG test should be performed to distinguish between neuromuscular junction disorders, channelopathies, and muscle disorders. If possible, a muscle biopsy is also advised. Lastly, a gene test is necessary to confirm the diagnosis.

Additional Tests or Key Results

Electromyography (EMG) test including needle EMG, routine nerve conduction tests, and repetitive nerve stimulation revealed normal. To confirm the diagnosis of muscle channelopathies, we performed a special EMG testing called the long exercise test, which measures the amplitude of compound muscle action potential (CMAP) for 50 min from a hand muscle that has been on a few minutes of exercise. No change of CMAPs was observed immediately after exercise. However, a continued decrease in amplitude reaches 76% at 50 min (Fig. 5.1b).

Molecular diagnosis revealed that both of the proband and her son carried a heterozygous mutation c.3716G>A (p.R1239H) in CACNA1S gene (Fig. 5.1c).

Discussion

Hypokalemic periodic paralysis (hypoKPP) is a rare channelopathy with a prevalence 1 case per 100,000 population, characterized by episodic paralysis with a concomitant hypokalemia. The paralytic attacks are reversible flaccid paralysis mostly leading to tetraparesis or paraparesis without respiratory muscles and heart involved. The weakness attacks were often triggered by rest following strenuous exercise, carbohydrate-rich meals, and cold temperatures. Acute paralytic crises may persist for a few hours or several days. The attacks may occur daily, weekly, monthly, or less often, even some patients have only one episode in life [1]. The disorder may be hereditary or caused by other factors including hyperthyroidism, Liddle's syndrome, renal tubular acidosis, alcoholism, hypothyroidism, Gitelman syndrome, gastroenteritis, and primary hyperaldosteronism [2].

Family hypokalemic periodic paralysis might be attributed to mutations in CACNA1S gene or SCN4A gene. CACNA1S and SCN4A encode the human skeletal muscle components of a calcium channel and the components of a sodium channel, respectively. The mutant CACNA1S and SCN4A alter the usual structure and function of calcium or sodium current density, which induced membrane depolarization. Membrane depolarization is followed by the inflow of potassium into skeletal muscle cells, disrupting regulation of muscle contraction, and thus leading to attacks of severe muscle paralysis [3–5].

In this family, the proband showed typically clinical features for hypoKPP, including episodic weakness trigged by rest following strenuous exercise, hypokalemia, positive exercise test of electromyography, as well as the mutations of CACNA1S gene. Treatment on this patient focused on relieving acute symptoms and preventing further attacks. The oral administration of potassium chloride is given incrementally to abort acute attacks. Nonpharmacological interventions that may be effective for preventing attacks include a low-carbohydrate diet and refraining from vigorous exercise. Some medications may help prevent attacks of weakness, included symptomatic potassium supplementation, potassium-sparing diuretics, and carbonic anhydrase inhibitors [6, 7].

5.2 Normal Potassium Periodic Paralysis

A 35-Year-Old Man with Repeated Spontaneous Paralytic Attacks in Proximal Muscles of Lower Limbs for 20 Years

Clinical Presentations

A 35-year-old man visited our hospital complaining of repeated spontaneous paralytic attacks predominantly proximal muscles of lower limbs for 20 years. The symptoms of weakness were precipitated by strenuous exercise, anxiety, and fatigue and lasted several days or longer. The frequency of episodes was less than 10 times per year. The patient was perfectly normal between the attacks. He had no major illness in the past and any addictions. His father and brother also had similar symptoms in their youth, but the severity and frequency of the attacks of his father relieved in his forties (Fig. 5.2a).

Neurological examinations revealed that cranial nerves were negative. The upper proximal muscle

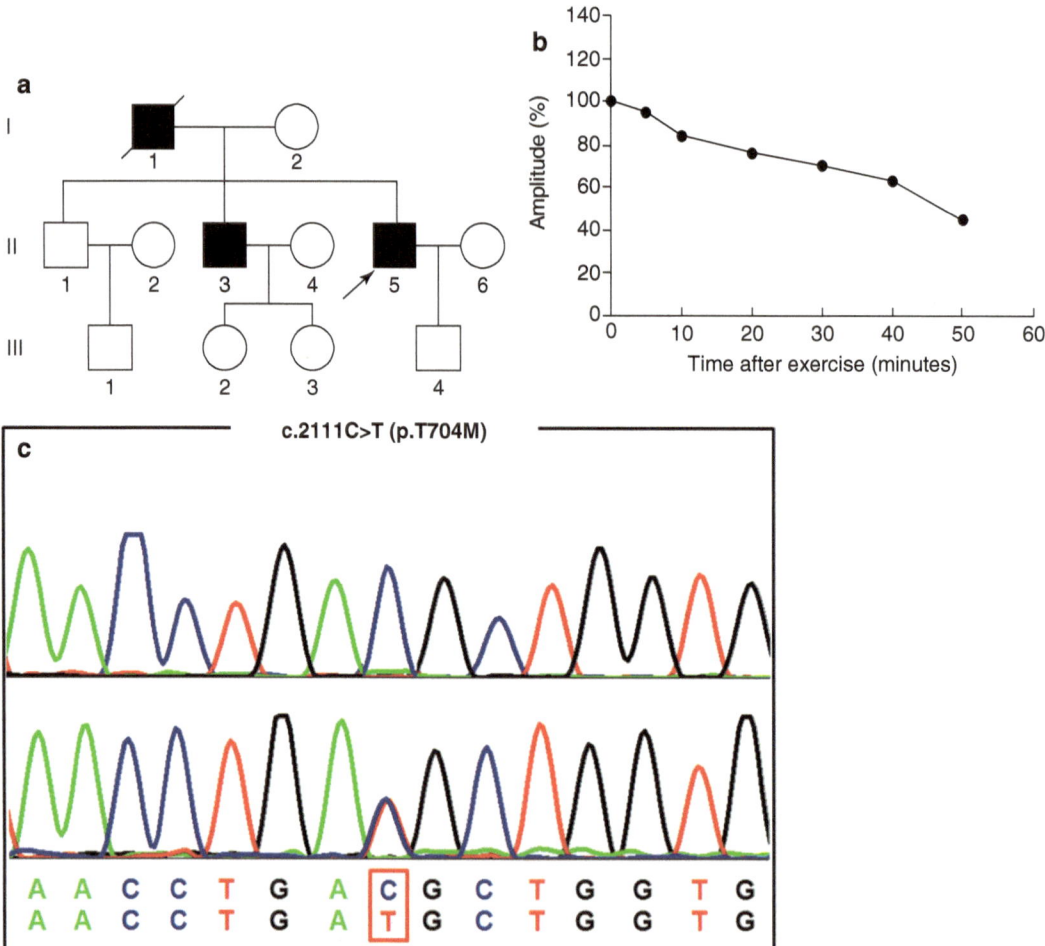

Fig. 5.2 (**a**) The patient's pedigree chart. *Arrow* indicates the proband. (**b**) Long exercise test showed amplitudes of CMAPs denoted as a percentage of its pre-exercise value are plotted against the time elapsed after hand muscle exercise. The results of CMAP amplitudes are noted as a percentage, where the 100% mean the CMAP amplitudes obtained during the pre-excise period. (**c**) Sequencing chromatograms showing the heterozygous T704M mutant in *SCN4A* gene. In the mutant sequence, the C-to-T transition at CDNA position 2111 results in the replacement of Cys by Met at codon 704

strength showed four grade in the lower limbs, and the distal limb muscle strength was normal. The muscular tension was decreased. Deep tendon reflexes were absent in all limbs. Babinski and Hoffmann signs were bilaterally absent. Deep and superficial sensation examinations revealed no deficits.

Laboratory investigations including potassium, calcium, magnesium, blood glucose, thyroid function, and creatinine kinase phosphate levels were within normal limits. ECG test was normal without arrhythmia.

Primary Diagnosis

The patient showed episodic weakness triggered by movement, emotional stress, and fatigue and lasted several days or longer. Neurological examination revealed flaccid weakness of proximal muscle in the lower limbs. These symptoms and signs hinted that the lesion must be situated in the spinal motor neurons, in the anterior roots, in a purely motor branch of a peripheral nerve, in the neuromuscular junction, or in the muscle itself. The differential diagnosis of a young patient with leg repeated spontaneous paralytic included spinal disease, Guillain-Barre syndrome, myasthenia gravis, and periodic paralysis. Spinal cord compression and vascular diseases were ruled out as there was no history of trauma and cardiovascular risk factors. Guillain-Barre syndrome was unlikely because the patient did not recount an ascending weakness and did not have a previous infectious disease. Myasthenia gravis was ruled out due to lacking of progressive fatigue. Familial periodic paralysis was suspected as the patient had remarkable family history.

Subsequently, an electromyography (EMG) test should be performed to distinguish between neuromuscular junction diseases and neurological muscle disorders. If possible, a muscle biopsy is also advised. Lastly, a gene test is necessary to confirm the diagnosis.

Additional Tests or Key Results

EMG tests were normal, including needle EMG, routine motor and sensory nerve conduction studies, and repetitive nerve stimulation. To confirm the diagnosis of muscle channelopathies, a specialized form of EMG examination called the long exercise test was performed. This test measures the amplitude of compound muscle action potential (CMAP) for 50 min following a few minutes of hand muscle exercise. After a long exercise test, no change of CMAPs was observed immediately. However, a decrease in amplitude appeared 5 min after exercise cessation, reaching its lowest 45% at 50 min (normal range <30%) (Fig. 5.2b).

Molecular diagnosis revealed the proband carried a heterozygous mutation c.2111C>T (p. T704M) in *SCN4A* gene (Fig. 5.2c).

Discussion

Primary periodic paralyses are hereditary disorders of ion channel dysfunction characterized by episodic flaccid paralysis. The disorder is classified as hyperkalemic periodic paralysis (HyperPP) or hypokalemic periodic paralysis (HypoPP) based on serum potassium level. Normokalemic periodic paralysis (normoKPP) is believed as a variant of hyperkalemic periodic paralysis [8, 9]. The clinical feather of normoKPP includes episodes of flaccid paralysis that are triggered by rest after exercise and usually last a few hours or infrequently days and attacks that may also be precipitated by anxiety and fatigue. Rarely respiratory and bulbar muscles will be involved in severe paralysis. Between attacks, myotonia can be elicited on examination in about 20–70% of patients [10].

Loss-of-function mutations in *SCN4A* are a well-established cause of disorders collectively termed sodium channelopathies, including HyperPP and normoKPP. *SCN4A* encodes the component of the skeletal muscle sodium channel mainly expressed in skeletal muscle. The most common are the missense mutations T704M and M1592V accounting for approximately 75% of affected individuals [10]. Homozygous *SCN4A* gene mutant mice showed muscle atrophy, limbs weakness, and abnormal muscle morphology [11].

In our family, the proband showed typically clinical features for channelopathies. The laboratory findings including normal serum potassium, positive exercise test of electromyography, and the mutations of *SCN4A* gene confirmed the diagnosis of normoKPP. The patient could benefit from sustained mild exercise after a period of more vigorous activity, high salt intake, and prophylactic use of the carbonic anhydrase inhibitor. It has been reported that acetazolamide reduced the frequency of attacks and may provide some relief from myotonia [12].

References

1. Abbas H, Kothari N, Bogra J. Hypokalemic periodic paralysis. Natl J Maxillofac Surg. 2012;3(2):220–1.
2. Santra G, De D, Sinha PK. Hypokalemic periodic paralysis due to proximal renal tubular acidosis in a case with membranoproliferative glomerulonephritis. J Assoc Physicians India. 2011;59:735–7.
3. Wang XY, Ren BW, Yong ZH, Xu HY, Fu QX, Yao HB. Mutation analysis of CACNA1S and SCN4A in patients with hypokalemic periodic paralysis. Mol Med Rep. 2015;12(4):6267–74.
4. Burge JA, Hanna MG. Novel insights into the pathomechanisms of skeletal muscle channelopathies. Curr Neurol Neurosci Rep. 2012;12(1):62–9.
5. Kim H, Hwang H, Cheong HI, Park HW. Hypokalemic periodic paralysis; two different genes responsible for similar clinical manifestations. Korean J Pediatr. 2011;54(11):473–6.
6. Sansone VA, Burge J, McDermott MP, Smith PC, Herr B, Tawil R, Pandya S, Kissel J, Ciafaloni E, Shieh P, Ralph JW, Amato A, Cannon SC, Trivedi J, Barohn R, Crum B, Mitsumoto H, Pestronk A, Meola G, Conwit R, Hanna MG, Griggs RC, Muscle Study G. Randomized, placebo-controlled trials of dichlorphenamide in periodic paralysis. Neurology. 2016; 86(15):1408–16.
7. Greig SL. Dichlorphenamide: a review in primary periodic paralyses. Drugs. 2016;76(4):501–7.
8. Venance SL, Cannon SC, Fialho D, Fontaine B, Hanna MG, Ptacek LJ, Tristani-Firouzi M, Tawil R, Griggs RC, investigators C. The primary periodic paralyses: diagnosis, pathogenesis and treatment. Brain. 2006;129(Pt 1):8–17.
9. Vicart S, Sternberg D, Fournier E, Ochsner F, Laforet P, Kuntzer T, Eymard B, Hainque B, Fontaine B. New mutations of SCN4A cause a potassium-sensitive normokalemic periodic paralysis. Neurology. 2004; 63(11):2120–7.
10. Miller TM, da Silva MRD, Miller HA, Kwiecinski H, Mendell JR, Tawil R, McManis P, Griggs RC, Angelini C, Servidei S, Petajan J, Dalakas MC, Ranum LP, Fu YH, Ptacek LJ. Correlating phenotype and genotype in the periodic paralyses. Neurology. 2004;63(9):1647–55.
11. Corrochano S, Mannikko R, Joyce PI, McGoldrick P, Wettstein J, Lassi G, Raja Rayan DL, Blanco G, Quinn C, Liavas A, Lionikas A, Amior N, Dick J, Healy EG, Stewart M, Carter S, Hutchinson M, Bentley L, Fratta P, Cortese A, Cox R, Brown SD, Tucci V, Wackerhage H, Amato AA, Greensmith L, Koltzenburg M, Hanna MG, Acevedo-Arozena A. Novel mutations in human and mouse SCN4A implicate AMPK in myotonia and periodic paralysis. Brain. 2014;137(Pt 12):3171–85.
12. Lehmann-Horn F, Jurkat-Rott K, Rudel R, Ulm Muscle C. Diagnostics and therapy of muscle channelopathies—Guidelines of the Ulm Muscle Centre. Acta Myol. 2008;27:98–113.

Muscle Diseases

Zhi-Qiang Wang and Wan-Jin Chen

Abstract

Myopathy is not one single disease but a general term used to describe a number of muscular disorders in which the muscle fibers do not function for many causes, resulting in common symptom of muscular weakness. Other symptoms, such as malaise, fatigue, atrophy and hyporeflexia, muscle cramps, stiffness, and spasm, can also be associated with myopathy. Myopathy in systemic disease is complex and has widely varying etiologies, including congenital or inherited, idiopathic, infectious, metabolic, inflammatory, endocrine, and drug-induced or toxic. So, muscle diseases can be subdivided as hereditary and acquired myopathies. The specific hereditary myopathies include muscular dystrophies, myotonic disorders, metabolic myopathies, periodic paralyses, and mitochondrial myopathies, while the acquired myopathies include inflammatory and endocrine myopathies. Important information to obtain during the patient's history includes family history, personal history, medications, and occupational and travel history. The following helpful laboratory tests may be used to evaluate patients with myopathy: creatine kinase (CK) levels with isoenzymes, levels of electrolytes, serum myoglobin levels, serum creatinine and blood urea nitrogen levels, thyroid function tests, antinuclear antibody levels, and genetic testing. Other additional studies may include: electromyography, electrocardiography, magnetic resonance imaging, and muscle biopsy. Because different types of myopathies are caused by many different pathways and etiology, treatments can range from supportive and symptomatic

Z.-Q. Wang (✉) • W.-J. Chen
Department of Neurology and Institute of Neurology,
First Affiliated Hospital, Fujian Medical University,
Fuzhou, China
e-mail: fmuwzq@sina.com

© Springer Nature Singapore Pte Ltd. 2017
Z.-Y. Wu (ed.), *Inherited Neurological Disorders*, DOI 10.1007/978-981-10-4196-9_6

management to therapy for specific conditions. Drug therapy, physical therapy, bracing for support, surgery, and massage are all current treatments for a variety of myopathies.

Keywords

Muscle diseases • Hereditary myopathies • Acquired myopathies • Etiology • Diagnosis • Treatment

6.1 Duchenne Muscular Dystrophy (DMD)

A 7-Year-Old Boy with Progressive Muscle Weakness and Calf Hypertrophy

Clinical Presentations

A 7-year-old boy was found to have progressive proximal muscle weakness of his lower limbs for 2 years. He was noticed to have difficulty in running or standing up after squatting since at the age of 5. Half year later, He developed to walk with waddling gait and was prone to fall down. He walked independently at the age of 6. Medical history revealed that he had delayed motor milestones. Family history (Fig. 6.1) disclosed that his elder brother developed the same symptoms at the age of 5 and lost the walking ability at the age of 11.

Neurological examinations revealed symmetric proximal weakness, which was more pronounced in lower limb and pelvic girdle muscles. The patient displayed tongue and calf hypertrophy. When he stood up from lying, he had to turn over to the ground and get up with the help of upper extremities.

The level of serum creatine kinase (CK) was found to be elevated to 18,517 U/L (normal range: 26–140 U/L). Serum alanine aminotransferase (ALT) and aspartate aminotransferase (AST) increased to 420 U/L (normal range: 0–40 U/L) and 180 U/L (normal range: 0–50 U/L), respectively. Electromyography (EMG) shows that weakness is caused by destruction of muscle tissue

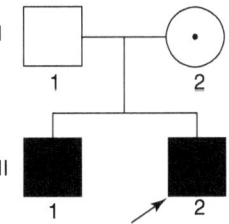

Fig. 6.1 Pedigree of the family. *Squares* indicate males; *circles* with a dot indicate female carrier; *the black symbols* indicate affected individuals; *the arrow* indicates the proband

rather than by damage to nerves. Both electrocardiogram and echocardiogram revealed unremarkable findings. Pulmonary function test showed a normal forced vital capacity.

Primary Diagnosis

This patient had progressive muscle weakness affecting predominantly the proximal lower limb and pelvic girdle muscles, prominent calf muscle hypertrophy, and significant elevation of serum CK since early childhood. All these symptoms and signs of the patient indicated the involvement of proximal skeletal muscle. EMG also provided objective evidence of myogenic damage. The long course of disease and family history implied that neurogenetic disease should be considered first for this patient. The extremely elevated CK level and prominent calf muscle hypertrophy hint the high possibility of Duchenne/Becker muscular dystrophy (DMD/BMD). The differential diagnosis includes polymyositis and other types of muscular dystrophy. Thus muscle biopsy and genetic analysis of *dystrophin* gene were necessary to verify the diagnosis.

Additional Tests or Key Results

A bicipital muscle biopsy revealed evidence of increased fiber size variation with moderate atrophy and hypertrophy. Inflammatory infiltrates were also found. Immunohistochemical studies revealed the expression of dystrophin was subtly reduced in most of muscle fibers.

Mutation of *dystrophin* gene caused by exon deletions or duplications was excluded by genetic testing performed by multiplex ligation-dependent probe amplification (MLPA) screening (Fig. 6.2a). Subsequently, the sequencing of *dystrophin* for point mutations revealed that both the patient and his affected brother harbored c.2852delT (p. ILE951ThrfsTer53) mutation (Fig. 6.2b). The further sequencing revealed the patient's mother also carried this mutation. Therefore, the patient was confirmed as DMD and prescribed with glucocorticoid for treatment, which may result in improvement of muscle strength and extension of ambulatory time.

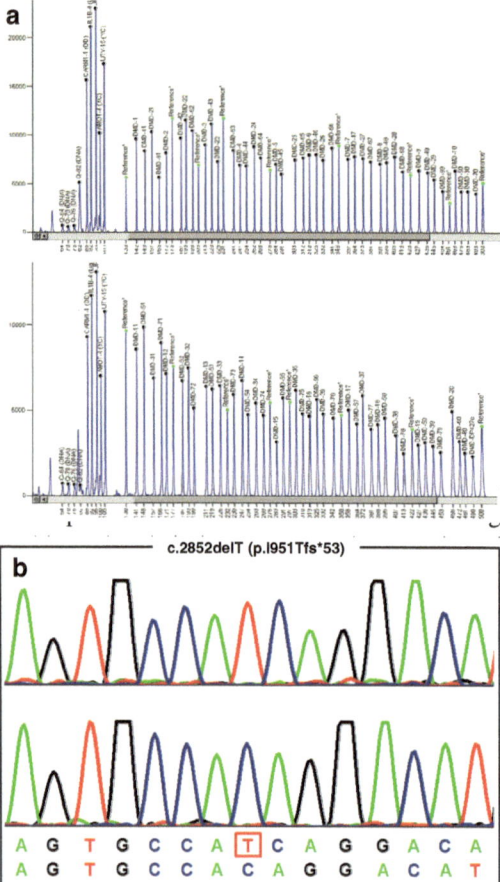

Fig. 6.2 Mutation analysis of the patient. (**a**) No deletion or duplication was found in 79 exons of *dystrophin* by multiplex ligation-dependent probe amplification (MLPA). (**b**) Chromatogram of c.2852delT mutation in *dystrophin*. The *upper panel* represents mutated sequence of the patient, whereas the *lower panel* is normal sequence of the control

loss of ambulation over 16 years and has better prognosis [1, 2].

The extremely high level of serum CK that can even be increased to 100-fold than normal level is a hint for DMD diagnosis. Myogenic damage confirmed by EMG is helpful in the differential diagnosis. A muscle biopsy can provide information on the amount of dystrophin and whether the protein is present. Differentiating total and partial absence of dystrophin also can help to distinguish DMD from BMD.

DMD/BMD is caused by mutations in the *dystrophin* gene located on the "X" chromosome. *Dystrophin* gene encodes a protein called dystrophin, which plays an important role in muscle contraction. Mutations in the dystrophin gene result in loss of dystrophin, leading to degeneration of muscle fibers. There are varied types of mutations in dystrophin gene, mainly including exon deletions, exon duplications, and point mutations. Because nearly 70% of the patients were found to have exon deletions/duplications of *dystrophin* [3], detection of deletions/duplications by MLPA should be firstly used for genetic test. If deletion/duplication testing is negative, then sequencing of *dystrophin* gene should be performed to look for point mutations.

To date, the main management of DMD includes pharmaceutical therapy and supportive treatment. For the ambulant patients, the use of corticosteroids has been confirmed to prolong ambulation by 6–24 months [4]. Corticosteroids may also help regarding respiratory function, cardiomyopathy, and scoliosis. However, corticosteroids use must be balanced against its side effects. After the patients lose walking ability, supportive treatment, such as nutritional support or cardiac and respiratory care, becomes more important than pharmaceutical therapy. Potential developments in gene therapy, such as exon skipping [5], bring hopes for future treatment of muscular dystrophy.

6.2 Lipid Storage Myopathy (LSM)

A 23-Year-Old Male with Muscle Weakness and Exercise Intolerance

Clinical Presentations

The patient, a 23-year-old male, was the first child of healthy non-consanguineous parents. He complained about progressive aggravated difficulty in walking and climbing since he was 10 years old. He often had premature fatigue and exercise intolerance, and sometimes accompanied by thigh and lumbar pain. His level of sports was poor at school. The symptoms could fluctuate or deteriorate under conditions of cold, fasting, infections, or intense activity. Due to the continuous elevation of serum CK (about 1000 U/L), a working diagnosis of polymyositis had ever been suspected, and standard prednisolone (initial 60 mg/day) therapeutic effect was transient and had unsustained improvement. Just a month prior to submission, he relapsed with increasing muscle weakness and myalgia with intermittent nausea and recurrent vomiting in the morning. One week ago, he completely lost the ability to stand up and had difficulty in raising his head. He had no deviation food habit. The perinatal and development history was uneventful. His 16-year-old sister had new-onset symptoms recently and began to suffer similar muscle cramps and poor physical fitness. But she had no antecedent muscle weakness of note (Fig. 6.3).

Neurological examinations revealed profound weakness of his neck, axial and proximal limb, and generalized muscle wasting. He presented a posture of dropped head when standing up and a waddling gait. Bilateral paraspinal muscles were mild atrophy (Fig. 6.4). Muscular tension was normal. Motor strength was symmetrical (MRCS, grades 0–5); neck strength was 2/5; deltoid and biceps brachii strength was 4/5; iliopsoas muscle strength was 3+/5; quadriceps femoris was 5/5; and distal limb muscle strength was 5/5. Sensory examination including pinprick, vibration, and position was intact. Tendon reflexes were reduced symmetrically and plantars down going. Cerebellar function was intact.

There was an obvious increase of muscle enzymes (serum CK 1100 U/L, normal <170 U/L;

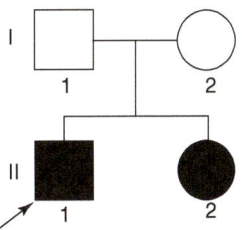

Fig. 6.3 Pedigree of the family with late-onset MADD. *Squares* indicate males, *circles* indicate females, *the black symbols* indicate affected individuals, *the arrow* indicates the proband

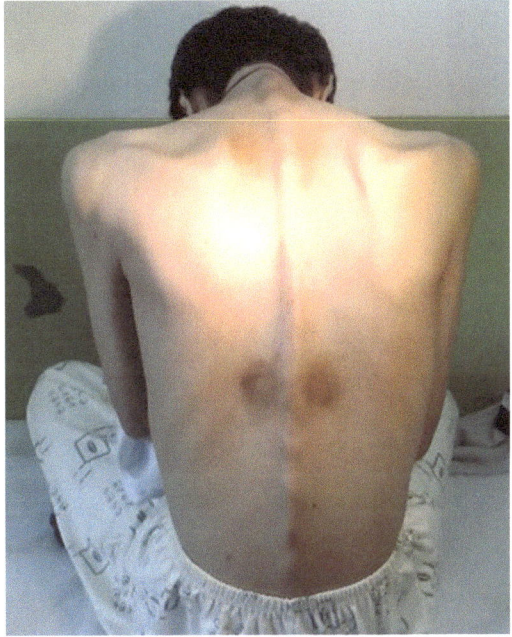

Fig. 6.4 Paraspinal muscles atrophy and neck muscle weakness (a posture of dropped head) of the patient

AST 78 U/L, normal <35 U/L; LDH 1156 U/L, normal <246 U/L). Resting blood lactate concentration is raised to 5.6 mmol/L (normal, 0.7–2.1 mmol/L). Routine blood parameters, renal profile, glucose, thyroid function, and inflammatory markers were normal. Electromyography (EMG) showed myopathic changes, while the nerve conduction and response to repetitive stimuli were normal. Pulmonary function was slightly reduced compared with predicted values (FVC 85% and FEV1 80%). Mild fatty liver was detected by abdominal ultrasound. Echocardiography showed no cardiomyopathy. Magnetic resonance imaging (MRI) of lower limb muscle exhibited diffuse atrophy accompanying fatty infiltration (Fig. 6.5). Brain MRI was normal.

Primary Diagnosis

The main symptoms and signs of the patient were progressive muscle weakness, exercise fatigue, and myalgia. The disease had a chronic and recurrent course from adolescence. Because of elevated muscle enzymes and myopathic changes in EMG and muscle MRI, the patient was primarily diagnosed with myopathies, including metabolic muscle diseases, limb-girdle dystrophy, or polymyositis. After reviewing the autosomal recessive form of pedigree, hereditary myopathies should be the prime consideration. So, the next step should be an operation of muscle biopsy for further differential diagnosis.

Additional Tests or Key Results

Hematoxylin and eosin (HE) staining revealed a remarkable variation in fiber size with small vac-uoles accumulating in biceps brachii muscle fibers (Fig. 6.6a). The oil red O (ORO) staining showed excessive lipid droplet accumulation in type 1 muscle fibers (Fig. 6.6b). No ragged red fiber was detected on MGT staining. A diagnosis of late-onset lipid storage myopathy (LSM) was made. Plasma carnitine, acylcarnitines, and uri-nary organic acid profiles using tandem mass spectrometry (MS/MS) and gas chromatography-mass spectrometry (GC/MS) are useful to make a diagnosis of type in LSMs. Urinary organic acid analysis demonstrated increased glutarate, 2-hydroxyglutaric acid, 3-hydroxyglutaric acid, glyceric acid, and 2-hydroxyadipic acid. Multiple elevation of short- (C6), medium- (C8, C10), and long- (C14) chain acylcarnitines were revealed by blood acylcarnitine analysis, which was consistent with the metabolic disturbance a mul-tiple acyl-CoA dehydrogenase defect (MADD).

Mutational analysis of the *ETF* and *ETFDH* genes from the patient revealed a compound

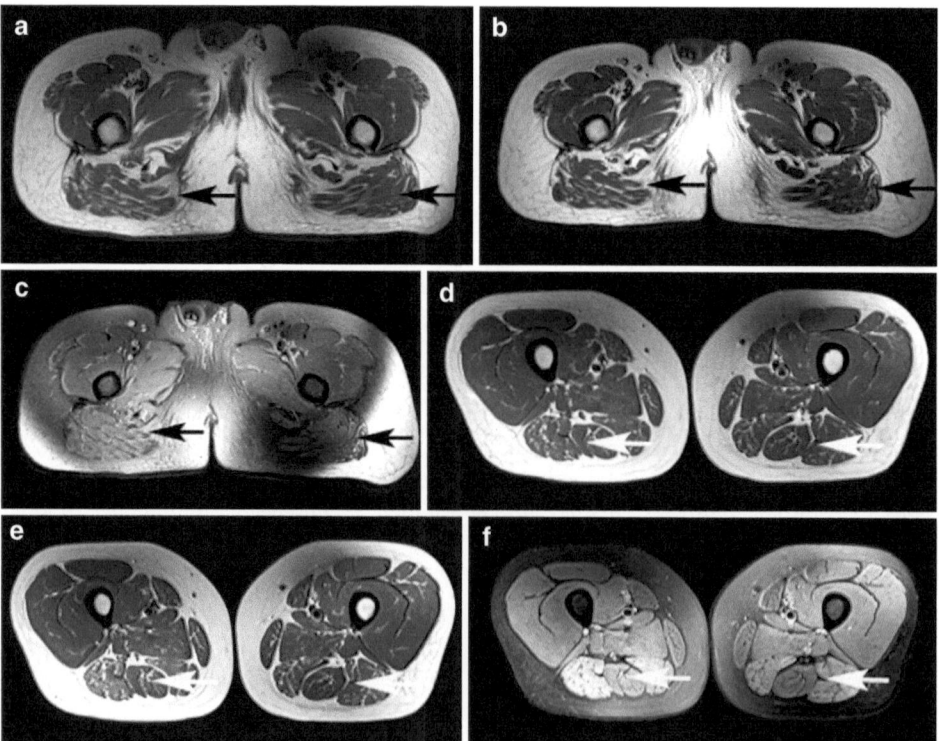

Fig. 6.5 Magnetic resonance imaging of lower limb mus-cle showed diffuse atrophy with fatty infiltration. T1-weighted images (**a**, **d**) and T2-weighted images (**b**, **e**) and fat suppression images (**c**, **f**) showed diffuse atrophy and mild fat infiltration of the gluteus muscles (indicated with *dark arrow*) and posterior thigh muscle group (indi-cated with *white arrow*) on horizontal scanning of pelvic (**a**–**c**) and thigh (**d**–**f**) level

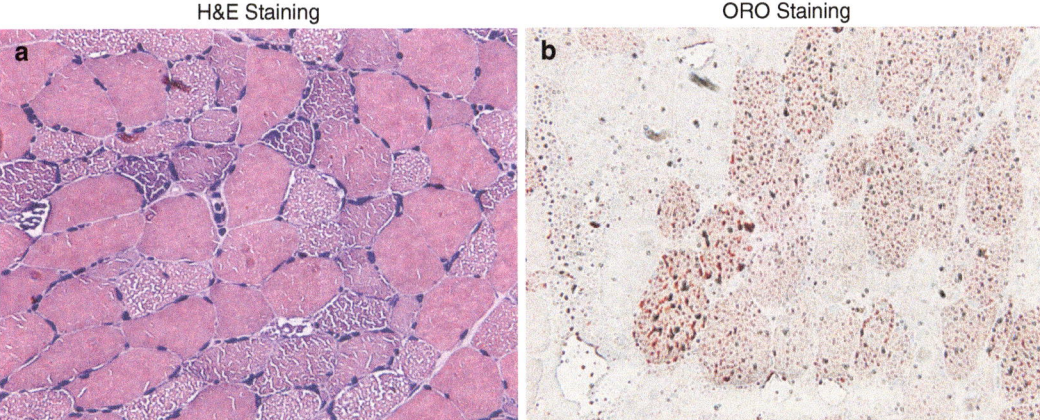

Fig. 6.6 Histological findings of (the left biceps brachii) muscle biopsy in the patient. (**a**) HE staining of muscle biopsy showing a marked variation in fiber size with small vacuoles accumulating in muscle fibers. Magnification, ×200 (**b**). The ORO staining showed excessive lipid droplet accumulation in type 1 muscle fibers. Magnification, ×200

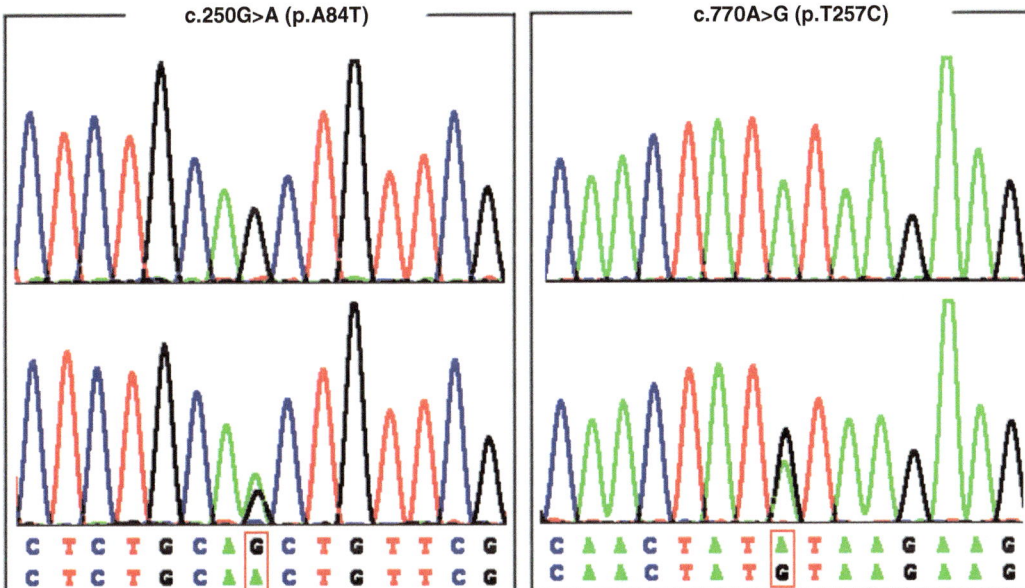

Fig. 6.7 Chromatogram of *ETFDH* mutations in the index patient. The compound heterozygous mutations c.250G>A (p.A84T) and c.770A>G (p.T257C) were con-firmed by Sanger sequencing. The *upper panel* of each chromatogram described the wild-type sequence, and the *lower panels* presented the heterozygous mutant sequence

heterozygous mutations of the *ETFDH* gene, c.250G>A (p.A84T), and c.770A>G (p.T257C) (Fig. 6.7). The mutations were inherited from each parent, c.250G>A (p.A84T) from his father and c.770A>G (p.T257C) from his mother. The gene sequencing for his younger sister showed the same heterozygous mutations.

Treatment and Following Up

He was immediately commenced on riboflavin 50 mg thrice daily, coenzyme Q10 10 mg thrice daily, and a diet of low fat, high-quality protein, and high carbohydrate. His muscle strength and exercise fatigue were associated with a steady improvement. Within 1 month, he was recovering with a normal motor strength and returned to normal daily life. The clinical blood biochemical indexes were returned to normal level. After 2 years of riboflavin commendation (the dose was reduced to 10 mg thrice daily), he was quite healthy with no muscle weakness or exercise intolerance. He got married and had a healthy baby.

Discussion

Through the above analysis, we presented a 23-year-old patient presenting with proximal muscle weakness, dropped head syndrome, premature fatigue, and increased levels of serum creatinine kinase and lactate initially. Muscle biopsy indicated LSM. Acylcarnitine profile showed an elevation of multiple acylcarnitines. Urinary organic acid analysis showed glutaric aciduria. Because of genetic findings and the good response to riboflavin treatment, the final diagnosis of riboflavin-responsive (RR-) MADD (OMIM 231680) can be established [6].

LSM is a general term which describes special types of metabolic myopathy characterized by lipid droplet accumulation in myofibers. Based on biochemical deficiencies and genetic causes, the syndromes are divided into four disorders: primary carnitine deficiency (PCD), multiple acyl-CoA dehydrogenase deficiency (MADD), neutral lipid storage disease with ichthyosis (NLSDI), and neutral lipid storage disease with myopathy (NLSDM) [7]. To make an accurate diagnosis, by specific laboratory tests including biochemical study and genetic sequencing, is very important for LSM as some of the types are clinically cured, such as this patient with late-onset MADD. This case also illustrates diagnostic difficulties that may arise and the importance of positive exclusion of metabolic disorders in such type of patients. MADD, also known as glutaric aciduria type II (GAII, OMIM 231680), could result in aberrant metabolism of fatty acids, amino acids, and sarcosine. It is an autosomal recessive disorder caused by defects in either electron transfer flavoprotein (ETF, encoded by *ETFA* and *ETFB*) or ETF-ubiquinone oxidoreductase (ETFQO, encoded by *ETFDH*) that transfer electrons from fatty acids to the respira-

tory chain [8, 9]. The deficiency of ETFDH is a major cause of RR-MADD, giving rise to reduced expression of ETFDH in muscle of ETFDH-deficient patients [6, 10–12]. Previous studies demonstrated three ETFDH hot spot mutations in China: c.250G>A (p.A84T) in patients from South China, and c.770A>G (p.T257C) and c.1227A>C (p.L409F) in those from both South and North China [6, 11, 12].

The phenotype of MADD is quite heterogeneous and classified as neonatal-onset forms with or without congenital anomalies, and later-onset form. In the neonatal-onset forms, patients usually die of serious metabolic crisis within a few weeks after birth. While the late-onset form is a mild form found in young and middle-aged with progressive or fluctuating proximal muscle weakness, exercise intolerance, and mild metabolic symptom such as vomit and oil disgusted [7]. This clinical phenotype is divided into pure myopathy and metabolism dominant. In this case, the main clinical features were symmetrical proximal limb and outstanding exercise intolerance. A valuable clinical clue to diagnose this disease may be the characteristic distribution of muscle weakness, especially the prominent neck involvement [10], which can also be called as dropped head syndrome. Meanwhile, the quadriceps femoris is mildly involved or normal, even in muscle histology [13]. For a subset of patients, the metabolism crisis is more prominent than myopathy, such as glycopenia, ammoniemia, hypotonia, encephalopathy, and cardiomyopathy [7]. In addition, most MADD patients have intermittent symptoms during the course, which deteriorated under several conditions of cold, fasting, or infections. However, the other chronic myopathy has no such clinical manifestations.

Routine laboratory tests frequently indicate mild to moderate elevation of serum muscle enzymes and lactic acid, except for accompany with rhabdomyolysis. EMG abnormalities are nonspecific. The diagnosis was based on elevated acylcarnitines and urine organic acids profiles using GS/MS which show corresponding abnormalities of fatty acids metabolism. But it often remains challenging, because the elevation of acylcarnitine levels may be mild and subtypical or detectable during acute metabolic crisis only [12]. Muscle MRI of lower limbs is a helpful tool in guiding clinical evaluation, because late-onset MADD patients show a typical muscle imaging pattern of fat infiltration and atrophy with posterior thigh muscle group and gluteus muscles involvement, while the anterior thigh group is sparing [14]. Therefore, the most effective way for definitive diagnosis is muscle biopsy and causing gene analysis. Muscle biopsy ORO staining could first narrow the differential diagnosis by revealing storage lipid in muscle fibers. The *ETFDH* gene is preferred screening gene for late-onset LSM. Mutation analysis revealed two mutations within *ETFDH*, c.250G>A (p.A84T) and c.770A>G (p.T257C). They are two impor-

tant hot spot mutations described previously in China, which could be employed as a fast and reliable screening method [6, 12].

Although the molecular mechanism of MADD is not well revealed, riboflavin (or vitamin B_2) supplementation (100–400 mg/d) has been known to strikingly reverse the clinical manifestations and metabolic profiles in RR-MADD patients [7]. While corticosteroids or carnitine alone did not result in a satisfying curative effect, riboflavin is a cofactor for ETF, ETFDH, as well as acyl-CoA dehydrogenases. CoQ10 supplementation has also been reported to improve muscle weakness and decrease the level of mitochondrial reactive oxygen species (ROS) in the patient cells [15].

6.3   Facioscapulohumeral Muscular Dystrophy (FSHD)

A 40-Year-Old Man with Progressive Weakness of Upper Arms and Shoulder Girdle

Clinical Presentations

The patient was a 40-year-old right-handed man who complained of presenting with progressive weakness and wasting of his shoulders and arms. His mother pointed out his lack of facial expression and unnatural smile at the age of 5. Meanwhile, he was noticed running with frequent falls compared with his peers. He developed inability to blow up a balloon and blow into a flute in his teens. He started to experience difficulties in lifting his right arm above the shoulder line and noticed scapular winging at the age of 18. Five

years later, he presented too much weakness and wasting of right upper arm to lifting heavy things. He had progressive difficulties in standing up and climbing up stairs since the age of 30. He denied diplopia or swallowing problems. His 63-year-old mother was examined neurologically and showed mild facial and both shoulder girdle weaknesses. His father was healthy.

The neurological examinations revealed moderate asymmetric facial weakness, marked shoulder girdle weakness and atrophy associated with bilateral scapular winging, and humeral weakness (Fig. 6.8). Manual muscle testing (MMT, 0–5 grade) showed asymmetric weakness of scapular and arm muscles (right 2–3 grade, left 4 grade) and proximal lower limb muscles (right 4 grade, left 5 grade); the distal extremities were 5 grade except for the left "drop foot." In addition, atrophy of pectoralis major, trapezius, and the

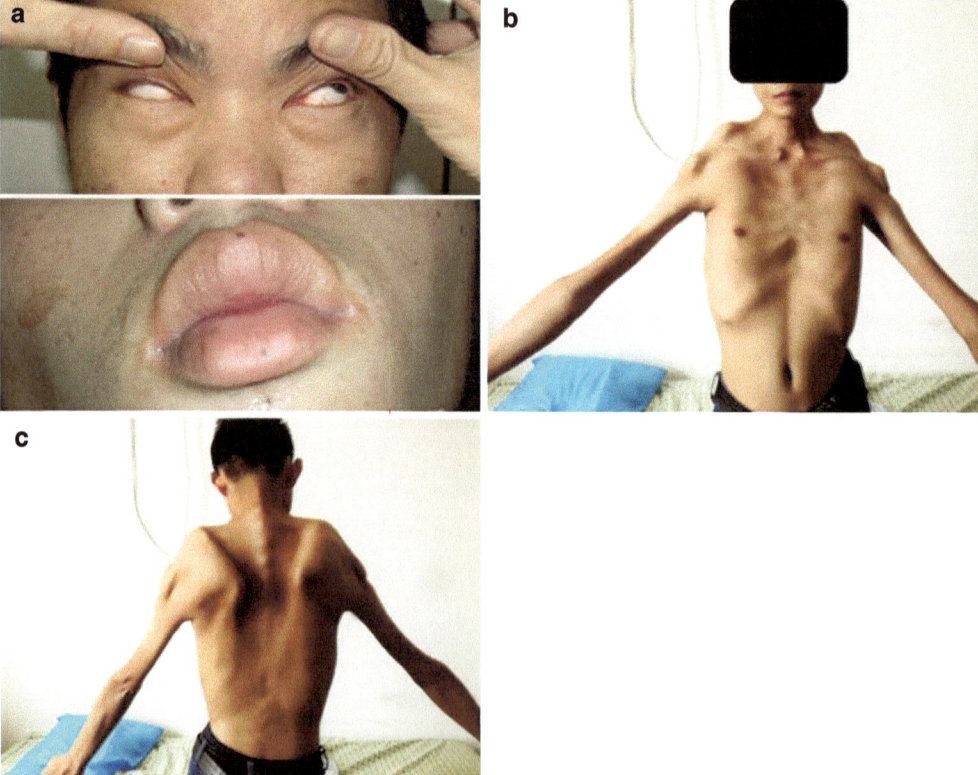

Fig. 6.8 Typical clinical manifestations in the patient with FSHD. (**a**) The appearance of asymmetric facial weakness of orbicularis oculi and oris showed incomplete eye closure and a fish-shaped upper lip. (**b**) Weakness and

atrophy of the humeral and pectoralis major muscle and involvement of the clavicular portion of the sternocleidomastoid muscle. (**c**) Marked winging of the scapula on active shoulder flexion or abduction

In Supine position

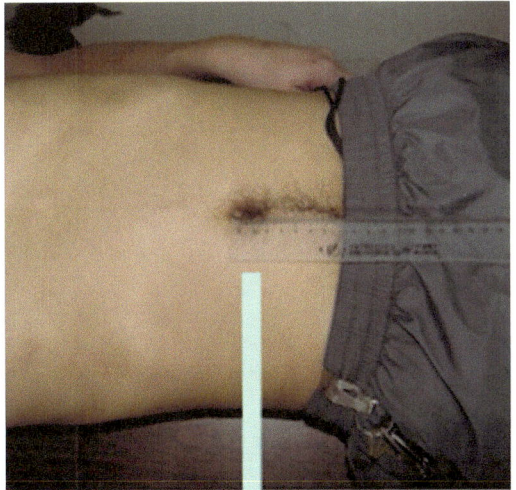

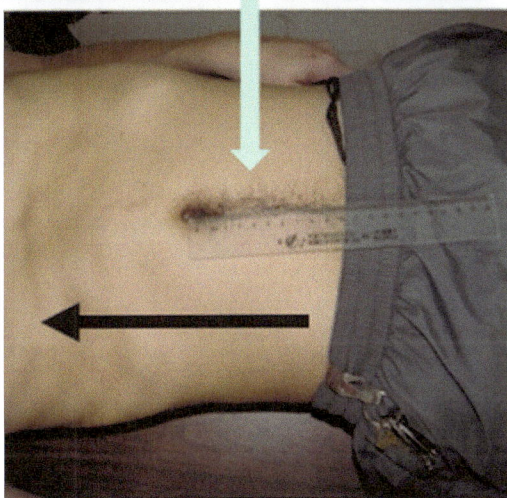

on flexion of the neck

Fig. 6.9 Beevor's sign. A marked upward movement of the umbilicus when the patient raised his head from a supine position

unilateral tibialis anterior muscles were noted. Beevor's sign (movement of the umbilicus toward the head with a flexion of the neck due to paralysis of the inferior portion of the rectus abdominis muscle, and the upper fibers predominate, pulling the umbilicus upward) was positive (Fig. 6.9). Arm tendon reflexes were obviously diminished. Coordination and sensory were normal.

His CK was mildly elevated to 246 U/L (normal <140 U/L). The nerve conduction studies of the ulna, peroneal, median, and sural nerves were normal. Electromyography (EMG) showed myogenic changes in the trapezius, deltoideus,

biceps brachii, and the unilateral tibialis anterior muscles. Muscle biopsy of biceps brachii revealed myopathic changes with the remarkable variation of fiber size, necrotic and regenerating fibers, and inflammatory cellular infiltration (Fig. 6.10). MRI examination assessed the asymmetric pattern and degree of involvement of the lower leg level (Fig. 6.11). Electrocardiogram (ECG) showed normal sinus rhythm. Respiratory function test showed mild respiratory abnormality.

Primary Diagnosis

The initial symptoms of this patient demonstrated the involvement of facial, shoulder girdle, and humeral weakness, with progressive development of the tibialis anterior muscle weakness. The evidence of myopathic damage from EMG and muscle biopsy supported the specific involvement of muscular system. Furthermore, the chronic course and autosomal dominant family history implies the possible diagnosis of hereditary neuromuscular disease, including facioscapulohumeral muscular dystrophy (FSHD), limb-girdle muscular dystrophy (LGMD), myotonic dystrophy (DM), and distal myopathy. However, the EMG of patients with DM often shows electrophysiological myotonic discharges. No distinctive findings of muscle biopsy could rule out DM and distal myopathy. The typical form of facial, shoulder girdle, and humeral weakness suggested the diagnosis of FSHD. It required genetic testing to distinguish FSHD from LGMD, although majority of the latter develop symmetrically.

Additional Tests or Key Results

Upon digestion with *EcoRI/HindIII* and *EcoRI/BlnI*, PFGE-based analysis of DNA demonstrated the presence of a 4q35-derived fragment of 22.0 kb (equate to six D4Z4 repeats) in the proband and her mother. Additional genetic testing disclosed a FSHD-sized 4qA-type allele in the patients, which was performed by using *HindIII* digested DNA hybridization with the 4qA and 4qB probes (Fig. 6.12). The molecular analysis finally confirmed the diagnosis of FSHD.

Discussion

FSHD (MIM 158900) is an autosomal dominant progressive neuromuscular disorder, and it is recognized as an epigenetic disease affecting

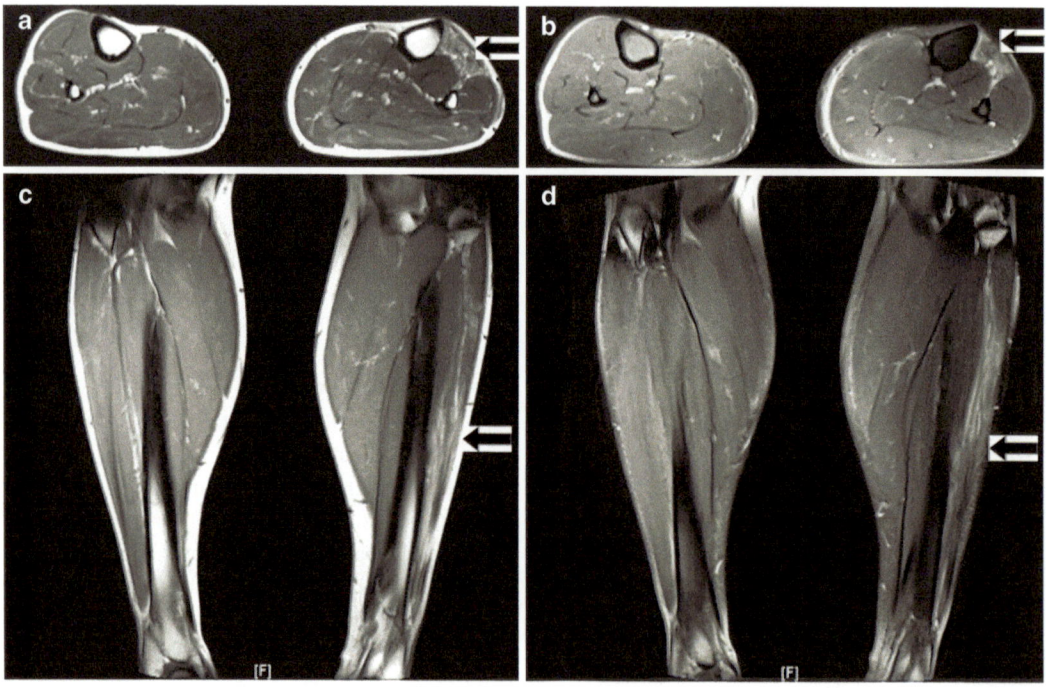

Fig. 6.10 MRI examination identified the asymmetric pattern and degree of involvement of the lower leg level. T1-weighted (**a**) and fat suppression images (**b**) showed distinct atrophy and dispersive fat infiltration (indicated with *arrows*) of the left mm. tibialis anterior and extensor digitorum longus on horizontal coronal scanning. The similar feature was showed on coronal scanning (**c, d**)

Fig. 6.11 Histological findings of (the left biceps brachii) muscle biopsy in the patient. There is remarkable variation of fiber size (*red arrows*). Interstitial areas with inflammatory cellular infiltration are visible (*black arrow*). Hematoxylin and eosin staining

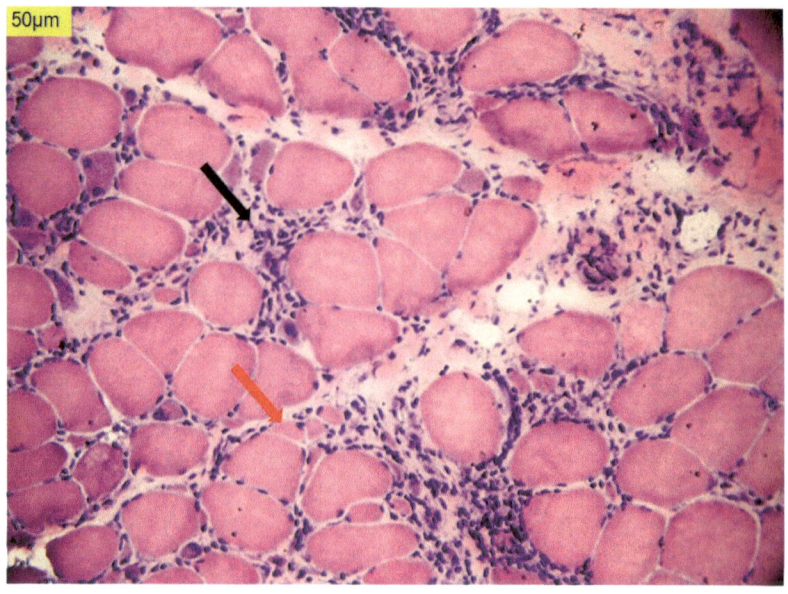

approximately 1:15,000 to 1:20,000 individuals. It is the third most common human muscular dystrophy, after Duchenne muscular dystrophy (DMD) and DM [16]. However, up to 30% of cases are sporadic, arising from de novo mutations. The classical FSHD syndrome, first

Fig. 6.12 Southern bolt analysis of digested-DNA fragment in the FSHD family using probes p13E-11 4qA and 4qB, separated by pulsed-field gel electrophoresis (PFGE). Genomic DNA was double digested with *EcoRI/HindIII* (E) and with *EcoRI/BlnI* (E/B), separated fragments by PFGE and hybridized them with p13E-11 (*left panel*). The proband (II₁) carried a 4q-type D4Z4 repeat array of 22.0 kb (*arrow*) inheriting from his mother (I₂). Then the same samples were digested with *HindIII* (H) and hybridized with probes 4qA and 4qB (middle and right). The corresponding 4q-type repeat arrays of 22.0 kb (*arrow*) were identified as 4qA variants. The size marker (*M*) indicated on the left is the MidRange PFG marker

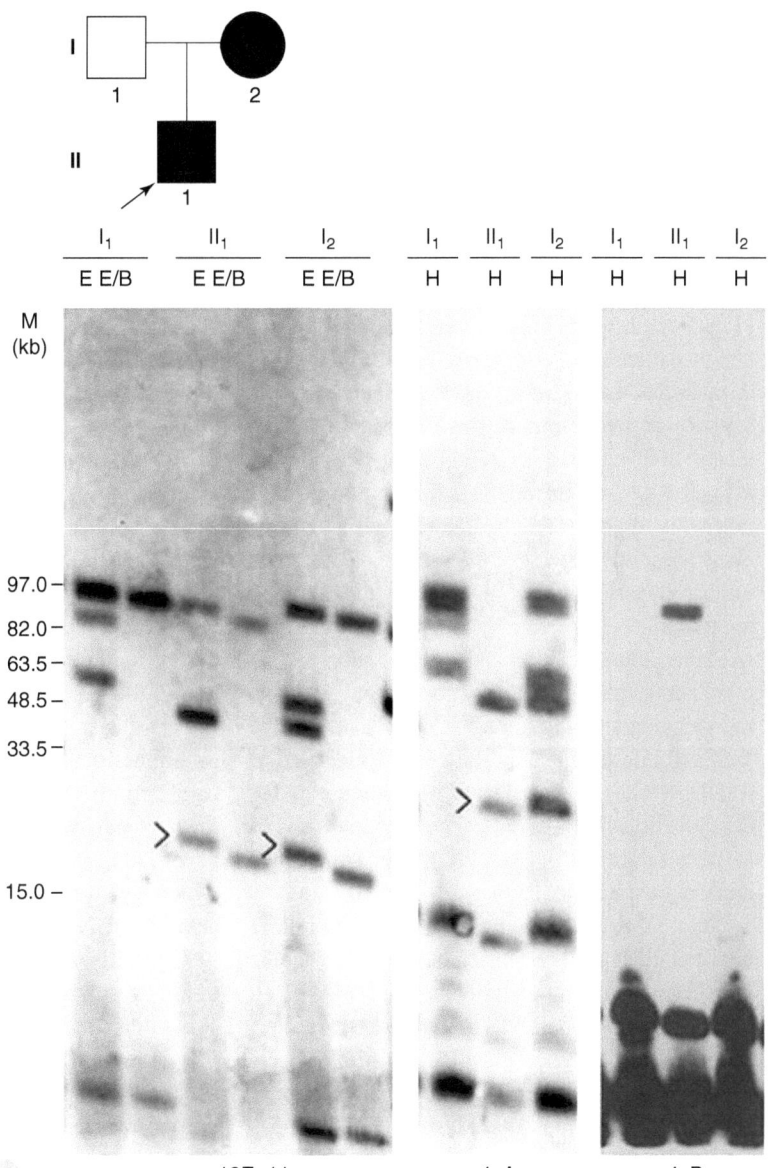

described by Landouzy and Dejerine in 1884, included the characteristic involvement of weaknesses and atrophy in skeletal muscles [17]. The FSHD phenotype usually develops in the second decade for most affected patients, but has been found to begin at any age widely ranging from infancy to late adulthood [16].

In most patients with FSHD, the clinical phenotype has been recognized to be distinctive. Weakness is often asymmetric and usually onset with asymptomatic facial weakness followed sequentially by the involvement the muscles of shoulder girdle and upper limb, finally spreading to lower extremity weakness with progression of the disease. The most commonly affected facial muscles are the orbicularis oculi and the orbicularis oris, which lead to difficulty in closing eyes, pursing lips, and transverse smile. Shoulder girdle and sternocleidomastoid muscles are also involved early associated with winging of the scapula when patients elevate the arms. The daily activities such as brushing teeth, washing face, combing hair, and lifting the arms over the head become difficult. The disease can gradually spread to abdominal, humeral, and lower extremity muscles. The weakness is often asymmetric, and this feature could distinguish FSHD from LGMD. High incidence of Beevor's sign was observed [18], which might especially help in the diagnosis of atypical cases. Cardiac evaluation showed abnormalities in approximately 5% of patients and commonly manifests as atrial arrhythmias, and rarely with conduction deficits [19]. Restrictive respiratory insufficiency requiring the use of a ventilator is rare in FSHD, occurring in about 1% of patients, and is delineated in association with severe affected patients, such as wheelchair dependence, severe kyphoscoliosis and lumbar hyperlordosis [20]. Besides the involvement of musculoskeletal system, the atypical extramuscular manifestation is referred to mental retardation, epilepsy, auditory impairment, and retinal vasculopathy that appeared mainly in patients with early onset [21–23]. The clinical spectrum of FSHD families exhibited large variation in the disease severity widely ranging from asymptomatic to severe disability [16]. However, the life expectancy appeared to be normal.

Serum CK levels are usually normal or mildly elevated. EMG shows mild to moderate myogenic damage pattern of motor unit potentials of involved muscles (small amplitude, polyphasic, and short duration). Histopathological analysis of muscle specimen often shows myogenic damage changes similar to other muscular dystrophies. DNA is referred to study for final confirmation if a physician considers FSHD as a high probability.

The molecular genetic basis of FSHD is complex. In patients with FSHD type 1 (FSHD1), accounting for 95% of FSHD patients, the genetic defect is associated with a heterozygous contraction of the tandem D4Z4 repeat array located at 4q35 subtelomeric region [24]. In normal individuals the D4Z4 repeat array is ranging from 11 units to 150 units, while patients carry less than 10 units, but at least there is 1 unit left [25, 26]. The pathogenic contraction requires occurring on a specific variant of 4qA distal to D4Z4 [27] (Fig. 6.13). Systematic studies demonstrated that the identification of D4Z4 residual repeats is helpful for predicting the patient's clinical severity, which is suggesting that more large D4Z4 repeats contraction tend to be associated with more severe phenotype as evaluated by the age of diagnosis and wheelchair dependence [28]. The pathogenic models of FSHD were proposed to relate with chromatin relaxation on D4Z4 contraction, which results in an epigenetic derepression of the *DUX4* retrogene embedded within the last D4Z4 repeat, and then participate in various pathways such as cell apoptosis, inflammation, and oxidative stress [29–31]. A small group of patients with FSHD2 have been identified to have *SMCHD1* mutations and the permissive 4 haplotype D4Z4 array together, which resulted in chromatin relaxation permissive for DUX4 expression [32].

Currently, there is no effective pharmacologic treatment for FSHD. Available studies demonstrate that surgical scapular fixation is an alternative intervention for improving some patients' life quality. Aerobic exercise appears to be potentially beneficial to patients with FSHD. Therefore, it is necessary for clinician to encourage patients' daily engagement of low-intensity aerobic actives or home-based exercise, without compromising muscle tissue [28].

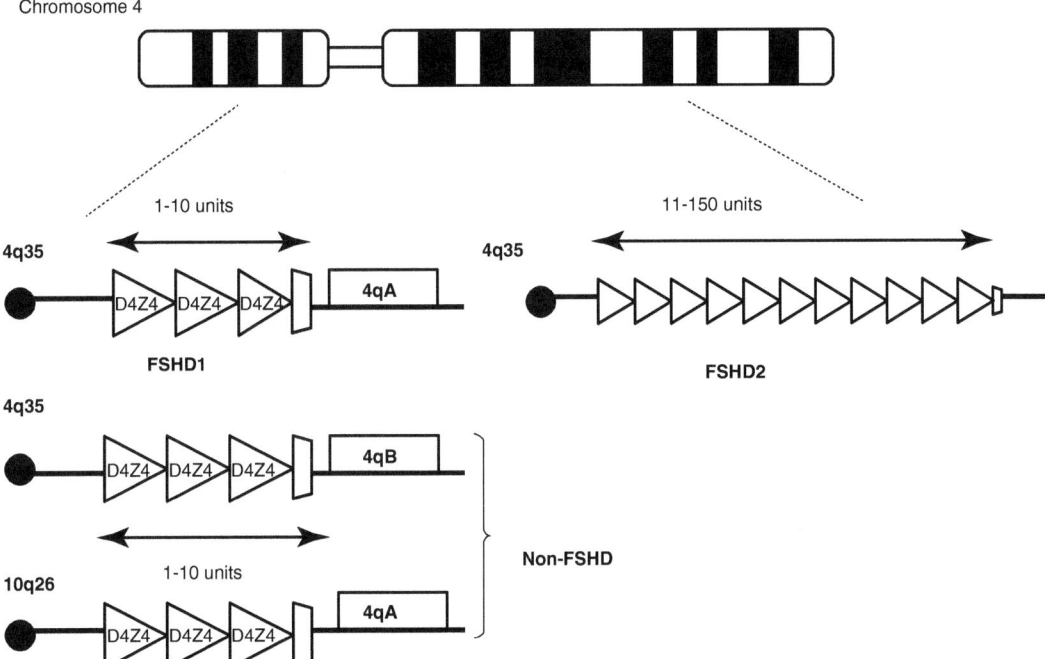

Fig. 6.13 Schematic representation showing the basic genetic background develop for FSHD. The regions of chromosome 4q35 and chromosome 10q26 have high sequence homology, and both contain the D4Z4 repeat array. Only contractions occurring on the permissive chromosomal background are associated with FSHD. Patients with FSHD1 have D4Z4 repeat of 1–10 units on chromo- somes 4qA. Although there are large region of homology between chromosome 4q35 and chromosome 10q26, D4Z4 contractions on 4qB or 10q chromosomes do not develop FSHD. Approximately 5% FSHD patients (FSHD2) have *SMCHD1* mutations and normal-sized D4Z4 repeats with permissive DUX4-PAS chromosomal background

6.4 Myotonic Dystrophy (MD)

A 29-Year-Old Man with Muscle Weakness and Myotonia

Clinical Presentations

A 29-year-old male complained distal muscle weakness and rigidity with difficulty in relaxation following strenuous muscle contraction ever since the age of 18. After that, he experienced progressive lower limb weakness, leading to easily tumble during his runs and climbs. At the age of 27, he showed symptoms of dysarthria, abnormal walking with foot drop, inability to lift heavy things, and deteriorative myalgia. He had no history of diabetes. He married for over 5 years without children. The family history was noteworthy that his father had similar symptoms and died with cardiac arrhythmia at the age of 68. His elder sister was in health (Fig. 6.14).

Neurological examinations revealed facial weakness and wasting, ptosis, droopy jaw, and the typical myopathic appearance (Fig. 6.15a). Neck extensor strength was 2/5 (MRCS, grades 0–5); iliopsoas muscle strength was 5$^-$/5; proximal muscle strength of lower limb was 4/5; and distal limb muscle strength was 3/5. He had difficulty in performing dexterity of the hands and foot drop. Grip and percussion myotonia were obvious (Fig. 6.15b). Palatal and pharyngeal muscles were also affected, causing problems of mild dysphagia and dysarthria. Deep tendon reflexes cannot be elicited. Impairment of light touch and pain sensation were not found.

The blood biochemical test revealed the slightly elevated level of serum creatine kinase (CK) 300 U/L (normal <140 U/L), and other indexes were normal. His renal and parathyroid function was normal. Electromyography (EMG) revealed myotonic discharge in affected muscles, which was suspected to be myogenic changes. The nerve conduction velocity was generally normal. Electrocardiogram (ECG) appeared conduction abnormity with right bundle-branch block. Magnetic resonance imaging (MRI) examination of the calf muscles showed that the affected muscles exhibited fatty degeneration (Fig. 6.16).

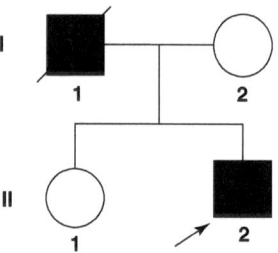

Fig. 6.14 Pedigree chart of the family. The *black field* indicates affected individuals, *circle* female, *square* male, *diagonal line* across symbol deceased, *arrow* proband

Primary Diagnosis

The major symptoms and signs of the patient were extensive myotonia and muscle weakness and wasting. In combination with the CK level and EMG results, the patient was diagnosed with myopathies. Furthermore, he showed chronic course of muscular disorder with family history, suggesting the tendency to hereditary myopathies. Based on the myotonic discharge in EMG, the diagnosis of myotonic dystrophy (DM) should be firstly considered. The differential diagnosis includes congenital myotonia, oculopharyngeal muscular dystrophy, and neuromyotonia. However, the patient with congenital myotonia often presents the intermittent muscle weakness without wasting of the affected muscles. The myotonic discharge of patient's EMG excluded the other diagnosis. Further examinations such as muscular histopathology, X-ray barium meal, the brain MRI, and the examination of slit lamp are necessary for the differential diagnosis.

Additional Tests or Key Results

X-ray barium meal revealed mild swallow restriction. The brain MRI showed mild focal white matter lesions (WMLs) in anterior temporal lobes with minor diffuse brain atrophy. Lens opacification was not detected by slit lamp. The pathological findings include myopathic changes with the variation in fiber size, numerous internal nuclei, sarcoplasmic masses, type 1 fiber atrophy, and type 2 fiber hypertrophy (Fig. 6.17), which implied the diagnosis of DM. Therefore, molecular analysis of myotonic dystrophy protein kinase (*DMPK*) gene was performed using the method of tri-primer PCR (TP-PCR). We

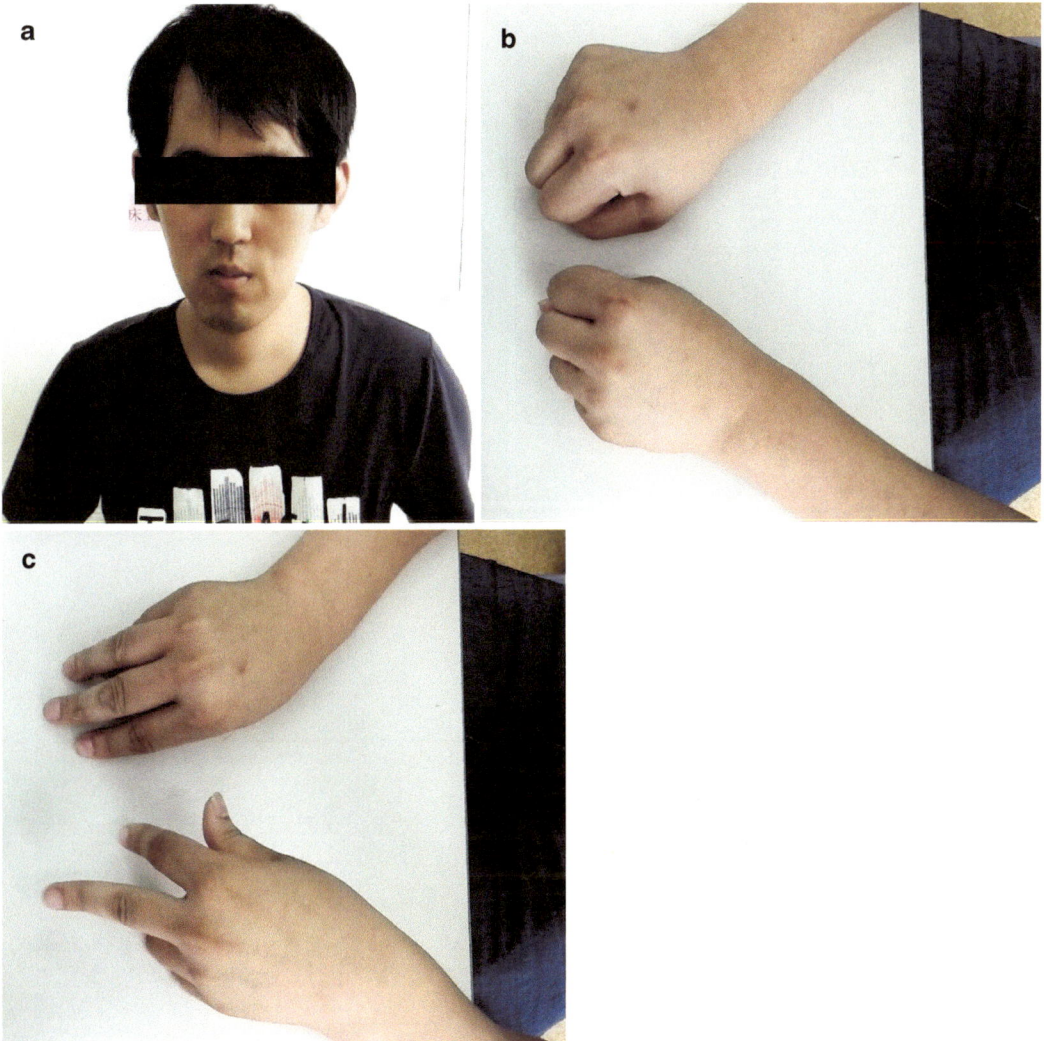

Fig. 6.15 Main clinical signs of the patient. (**a**) Facial weakness and wasting gave rise to the typical myopathic appearance (or "hatchet" appearance) of hollow cheeks and droopy jaw. (**b**) *Left*: Clasped hands of the patient. *Right*: Unclasping of the hands was delayed, exhibiting the myotonic phenomenon. (**c**) Patient has difficulty in relax his hands after making a fist

found that the patient carried a pathogenic cytosine-thymine-guanine (CTG) triplet repeats expansion in *DMPK* gene (Fig. 6.18), which finally confirmed the diagnosis of DM1.

Discussion

DM is the most common muscular dystrophy in adult, which is divided into two distinct forms of DM type 1 (DM1, Steinert's disease) and DM type 2 (DM2) based on the clinical features and genetic differences. Both of them are autosomal dominant, multisystemic diseases with a core pattern of clinical features including prominent myotonia, progressive wasting and weakness of skeletal muscle, cardiac conduction defects, cataracts, and endocrine disorders [33].

DM1 has first been described as a "classic" type of myotonic dystrophy with a prevalence of about 1/8000 people worldwide. Its onset can be congenital, juvenile, adult, or late. In this case, our adult-onset patient was characterized for distal muscular dystrophy and myotonia, which mani-

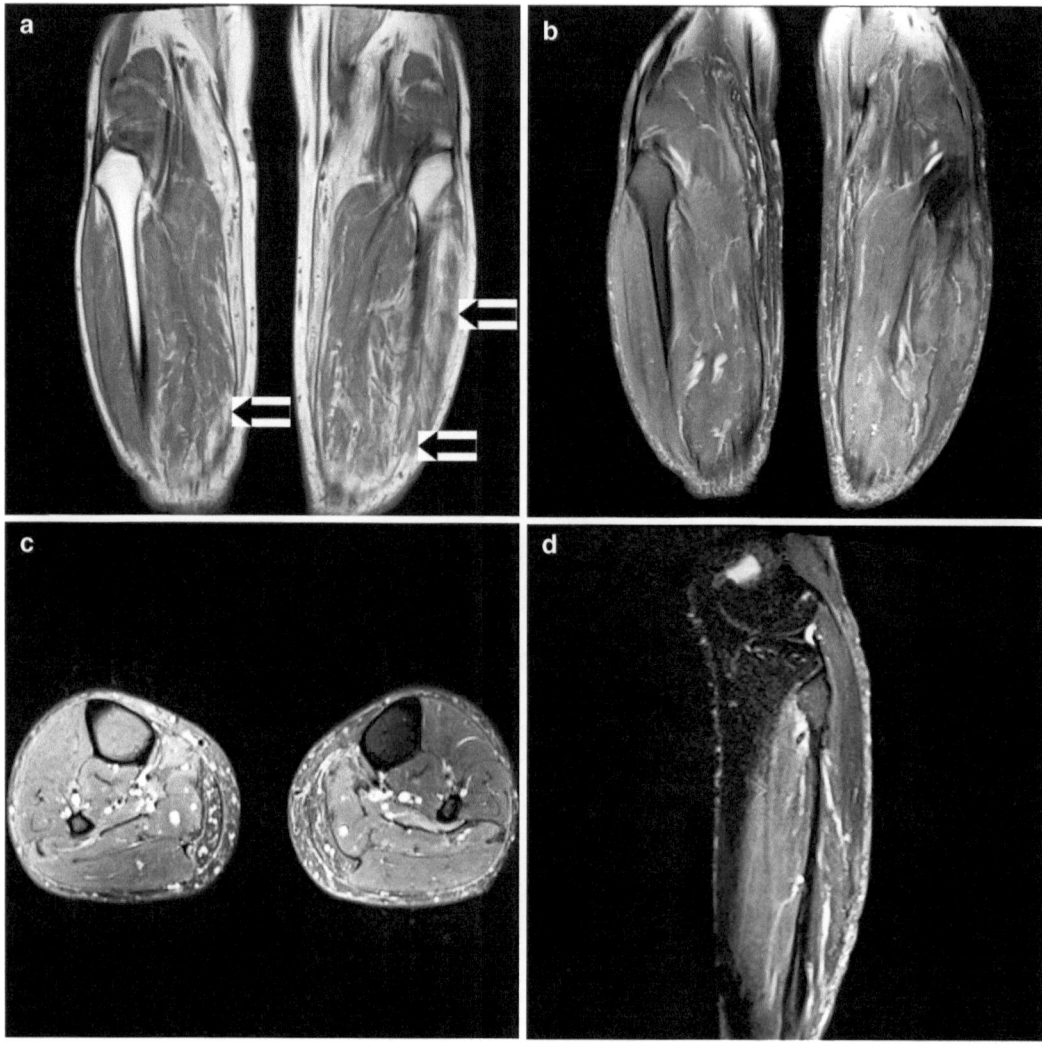

Fig. 6.16 MRI examination of the calf muscles showed fatty degeneration and mild atrophy. T1-weighted (**a**) and fat suppression images (**b**) showed dispersive fat infiltration (indicated with *arrows*) of the calf muscles on coronal scanning. Fat suppression images showed mild atrophy of the calf muscles on horizontal (**c**) and anteroposterior axes (**d**) scanning

fested as a delayed relaxation voluntary contraction of skeletal muscle. Especially, grip myotonia is his initial symptom preceding the presentation of muscle weakness. The myotonia may frequently improve by repeated muscle contraction, called the "warm-up phenomenon." Due to facial weakness and wasting, many patients exhibit atypical facial appearance, including ptosis of the upper eyelid, turn V-shaped upper lip (also known as a tent- or fish-shaped upper lip), or "hatchet" appearance. It should be carefully differentiated

from facioscapulohumeral muscular dystrophy (FSHD) for the similar facial symptoms. Another common feature is frontal balding. The myotonia involvements of tongue, pharyngeal, and palatal muscles weakness often cause indistinct speech and dysarthria [34]. In this case, the patient showed hollow cheeks and drooping jaw, which suggest the weakness and wasting of masticatory and temporal muscles, as well as neck flexors weakness and early involvement of long finger flexors. Ankle dorsiflexion weakness can result in frequent

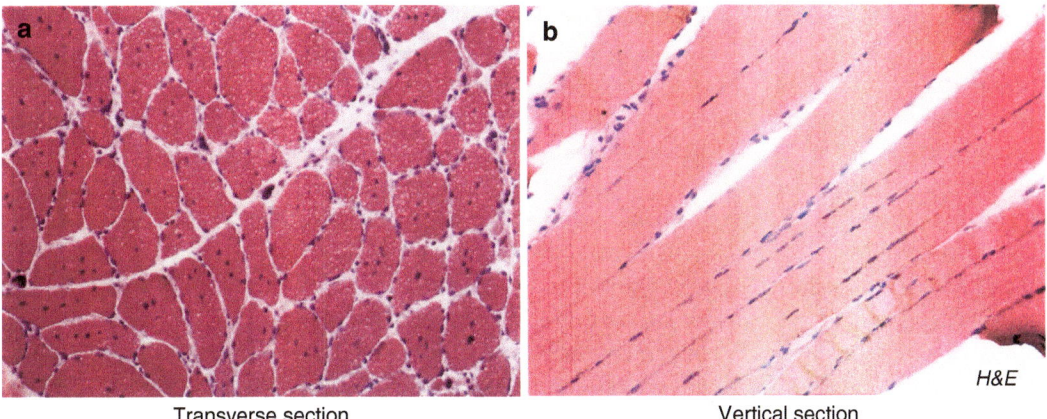

Transverse section   Vertical section

Fig. 6.17 Histological findings of (the left biceps brachii) muscle biopsy in the patient. (**a**) The transverse section of muscle specimen showed the variation in fiber size, numerous internal nuclei, and sarcoplasmic masses. (**b**) The vertical section of muscle specimen showed internal nuclei located in longitudinal chains. Hematoxylin and eosin staining; magnification, ×200

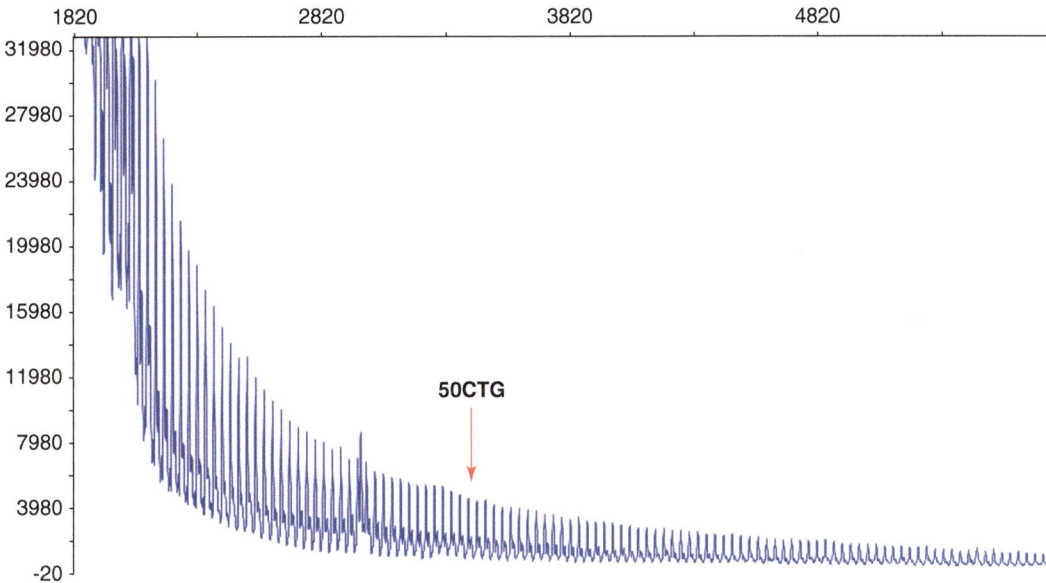

Fig. 6.18 TP-PCR analysis of *DMPK* gene in the patient. In normal individuals, the number of CTG repeats in the *DMPK* gene is ranging from 5 to 37; the patient was detected to have more than 50 CTG repeats by TP-PCR analysis

falls. Although suffering from distal muscle weakness with slowly progressive, the proximal muscles of DM1 patients are affected later in clinical course.

The extra-muscular clinical manifestations mainly including: cardiac abnormality, respiratory failure, endocrine problems, cataracts, neuropsychological, and cognitive impairments [35].

Cardiac conduction disease is common in DM1 and is the primary cause of disease morbidity and mortality. Conduction disturbances and tachyarrhythmias, such as malignant arrhythmia and progressive left ventricle dysfunction, may result in sudden death. Dilated cardiomyopathy is observed among some patients. Respiratory insufficiency is caused by the weakness of respiratory muscle, especially involvement of diaphragm. Respiratory failures can easily occur with aspiration pneumonia secondary to swallowing problems. Neuropsychological deficits and cognitive impairment have been frequently documented and significantly impact on life quality for patients and families [36, 37]. Nocturnal apneic episodes and excessive daytime sleepiness (EDS) are common manifestations. Posterior subcapsular cataracts develop in most patients, and some of them present cataract during youth without any other symptom. Gastrointestinal symptoms are frequent in DM1 and caused by the involvement of smooth muscle with dysphagia, emesis, episodic diarrhea, and more. Finally, endocrine abnormalities cover disturbances of the thyroid, gonads, as well as hypothalamus and pancreas, the latter associated with insulin resistance. Testicular atrophy results in infertility in some of male patients, while menstrual irregularities and habitual abortion are common in female patients.

Laboratory examinations sometimes reveal mild increased serum CK. EMG evidence of myotonia was an important marker before the genetic testing became available. The distal muscles and musculus facialis are often detected with myotonic discharges and myopathic pattern. Histological findings of muscle biopsy in symptomatic patients are always abnormal, and sufficiently characteristic that a diagnosis of DM can be referenced to muscle biopsy. The features of affected muscles include numerous of internal nuclei, increased variation in fiber size, fibrosis, sarcoplasmic masses, ring fibers, early type I fiber atrophy, and type II fiber hypertrophy. The brain MRI often shows brain atrophy and increasing white matter signals with T2-weighted images [38].

DM1 is caused by an expansion of unstable CTG trinucleotide repeat in the 3′-untranslated region (UTR) of the *DMPK* gene located on chromosome 19q13.3, which codes a myosin kinase expressed in skeletal muscle [39, 40]. In normal individuals, the number of CTG repeats ranges from 5 to 37, while the pathogenic expansion of CTG repeats is over 50. The mutation is associated with mis-splicing of mRNA species which affect many cellular processes in multiple organs [41]. The patients with CTG repeats expansion ranging between 38 and 49 are usually clinically asymptomatic, but their offspring are at risk of having larger pathologically expanded repeats. The symptomatic patient with DM1 often carries more than 50 CTG repeats, ranging from 50 to 4000. There is not a clear correlation between the phenotype and genetic repeats number. The children with DM1 may present a larger repeat numbers than the transmitting parents. The phenomenon of CTG repeat instability in parent-offspring causes anticipation and increases clinical severity and early-onset age in successive generations [42]. A child presents congenital DM1 with increasing CTG repeats number usually with maternal transmission, while the paternal inheritance patients are rarely reported.

DM2 is described as proximal myotonic myopathy and shares many clinical features of DM1. So DM2 is a multisystem disorder and the leading symptoms are myotonia and muscle weakness. There are several differences between DM1 and DM2 [33, 35]. First, the onset age of DM2 is much later than DM1, often in the third decade. Second, DM2 patients have more severe stiffness, myalgia, and fatigue than those with DM1. Third, DM2 patients are present with proximal muscles during the early course, while DM1 patients show mildly affected. The extra-muscular symptoms are also common in DM2. In DM2, laboratory examinations usually show the high level of serum cholesterol. EMG shows myotonic discharges in proximal limb muscles. Histological analysis reveals that multiple internal nuclei and fiber size variation primarily involved type 2 muscle fibers and numerous nuclear clumps as well.

DM2 caused by an unstable tetranucleotide repeat expansion, CCTG, in intron 1 of the nucleic acid-binding protein (*CNBP*) gene (also known as zinc finger 9 gene, *ZNF9*) located on chromosome 3q21 [43]. The size of the CCTG repeat is less than 30 repeats in normal individuals while the range of the expansion repeats number in DM2 is huge. The large repeat expansion for DM2 is ranging from 75 to11000. Unlike DM1, there is no correlation between CCTG repeats expanded size and onset age or phenotype in DM2.

In spite of the clinical and genetic similarities, DM1 and DM2 are distinct disorders requiring different diagnostic and management strategies. DM1 is classified in four different forms: congenital, early childhood, adult onset, and late onset. Congenital form is the most severe one and characterized by extreme muscle weakness and mental retardation. While the phenotype in DM2 is hypervariable, there are no distinct clinical subgroups. In contrast to DM1, myotonic discharges may be absent even on EMG in some DM2 patients. Consequently, a large proportion of DM2 patients remain underdiagnosed. The long delayed diagnosis may cause unnecessary problems for the patients' lives management, uncertain prognosis, and treatment. As a genetic disease, the DM diagnostic method is mutation verification by genetic tests. In DM1, clinical manifestations, family history, and the results of assistant examinations are often provided distinctive proofs for clinical diagnosis, and the mutation can be confirmed by PCR or southern blot analysis. Furthermore, TP-PCR has come into routine diagnostic process which represents a simple and reliable way that can rapidly identify the presence of expanded alleles for disorders caused by repeat expansions, although it cannot provide accurate numbers of repeat sequences [44]. On the contrary, conventional PCR and southern blot analysis are not adequate for a defined molecular diagnosis in DM2 since the extremely large of the expansion mutation. Several highly sensitive and specific methods have been developed for DM2 mutation verification including a complex genotyping diagnostic procedure, long-range PCR, and a tetraplet PCR.

Although there is no curative therapy for DM, active management includes careful evaluation and monitoring possible complications [33]. For patients with cardiorespiratory disorders, active monitoring, lower threshold for input, and long-term follow-up are necessary. Early treatment of sleep-related disordered breathing with nocturnal noninvasive mechanical ventilation is a preferential consideration. Insulin resistance becomes a problem which patients needs more insulin or other medicines to control glucose level. Antimyotonia therapy is helpful for the patients associated with frequent and persistent muscle stiffness and pain. Some individuals are in response to mexiletine or carbamazepine. Evidence showed that mexiletine of 150–200 mg thrice daily is effective and safe for improving myotonia [45].

References

1. Bushby K, Finkel R, Birnkrant DJ, et al. Diagnosis and management of Duchenne muscular dystrophy, part 1: diagnosis, and pharmacological and psychosocial management. Lancet Neurol. 2010;9:77–93.
2. Bushby K, Finkel R, Birnkrant DJ, et al. Diagnosis and management of Duchenne muscular dystrophy, part 2: implementation of multidisciplinary care. Lancet Neurol. 2010;9:177–89.
3. Chen WJ, Lin QF, Zhang QJ, He J, Liu XY, Lin MT, et al. Molecular analysis of the dystrophin gene in 407 Chinese patients with Duchenne/Becker muscular dystrophy by the combination of multiplex ligation-dependent probe amplification and sanger sequencing. Clin Chim Acta. 2013;423:35–8.
4. Manzur AY, Kuntzer T, Pike M, Swan A. Glucocorticoid corticosteroids for Duchenne muscular dystrophy. Cochrane Database Syst Rev. 2008;23: CD003725.
5. Kole R, Krieg AM. Exon skipping therapy for Duchenne muscular dystrophy. Adv Drug Deliv Rev. 2015;87:104–7.
6. Wang ZQ, Chen XJ, Murong SX, Wang N, Wu ZY. Molecular analysis of 51 unrelated pedigrees with late-onset multiple acyl-CoA dehydrogenation deficiency (MADD) in southern China confirmed the most common ETFDH mutation and high carrier frequency of c.250G>A. J Mol Med. 2011;89(6): 569–76.
7. Liang WC, Nishino I. Lipid storage myopathy. Curr Neurol Neurosci Rep. 2011;11(1):97–103.
8. Schiff M, Froissart R, Olsen RK, Acquaviva C, Vianey-Saban C. Electron transfer flavoprotein deficiency: functional and molecular aspects. Mol Genet Metab. 2006;88(2):153–8.
9. Ohkuma A, Noguchi S, Sugie H, Malicdan MC, Fukuda T, Shimazu K, López LC, Hirano M, Hayashi YK, Nonaka I, Nishino I. Clinical and genetic analysis of lipid storage myopathies. Muscle Nerve. 2009;39(3):333–42.
10. Olsen RK, Olpin SE, Andresen BS, Miedzybrodzka ZH, Pourfarzam M, Merinero B, Frerman FE, Beresford MW, Dean JC, Cornelius N, Andersen O, Oldfors A, Holme E, Gregersen N, Turnbull DM, Morris AA. ETFDH mutations as a major cause of riboflavin-responsive multiple acyl-CoA dehydrogenation deficiency. Brain. 2007;130(Pt 8):2045–54.
11. Wen B, Dai T, Li W, Zhao Y, Liu S, Zhang C, Li H, Wu J, Li D, Yan C. Riboflavin responsive lipid storage

myopathy caused by ETFDH gene mutations. J Neurol Neurosurg Psychiatry. 2010;81(2):231–6.

12. Xi J, Wen B, Lin J, Zhu W, Luo S, Zhao C, Li D, Lin P, Lu J, Yan C. Clinical features and ETFDH mutation spectrum in a cohort of 90 Chinese patients with late-onset multiple acyl-CoA dehydrogenase deficiency. J Inherit Metab Dis. 2014;37:399–404.

13. Fu HX, Liu XY, Wang ZQ, Jin M, Wang DN, He JJ, Lin MT, Wang N. Significant clinical heterogeneity with similar ETFDH genotype in three Chinese patients with late-onset multipleacyl-CoA dehydrogenase deficiency. Neurol Sci. 2016;37(7): 1099–105.

14. Liu XY, Jin M, Wang ZQ, Wang DN, He JJ, Lin MT, Fu HX, Wang N. Skeletal muscle magnetic resonance imaging of the lower limbs in late-onset lipid storage myopathy with electron transfer flavoprotein dehydrogenase gene mutatins. Chin Med J. 2016;129(12): 1425–31.

15. Cornelius N, Byron C, Hargreaves I, Guerra PF, Furdek AK, Land J, Radford WW, Frerman F, Corydon TJ, Gregersen N, Olsen RK. Secondary coenzyme Q10 deficiency and oxidative stress in cultured fibroblasts from patients with riboflavinresponsive multiple Acyl-CoA dehydrogenation deficiency. Hum Mol Genet. 2013;22(19):3819–27.

16. Patberg, G.W. (1982). Facioscapulohumeral disease. PhD thesis, Leiden University, Leiden.

17. Landouzy L, Dejerine J. De la myopathie atrophique progressive. Rev Med Fr. 1885;98:53–5.

18. Eger K, Jordan B, Habermann S, Zierz S. Beevor's sign in facioscapulohumeral muscular dystrophy: an old sign with new implications. J Neurol. 2010; 257(3):436–8.

19. Laforet P, de Toma C, Eymard B, et al. Cardiac involvement in genetically confirmed facioscapulohumeral muscular dystrophy. Neurology. 1998;51(5):1 454–6.

20. Wohlgemuth M, van der Kooi EL, van Kesteren RG, et al. Ventilatory support in facioscapulohumeral muscular dystrophy. Neurology. 2004;63(1):176–8.

21. Lutz KL, Holte L, Kliethermes SA, Stephan C, Mathews KD. Clinical and genetic features of hearing loss in facioscapulohumeral muscular dystrophy. Neurology. 2013;81(16):1374–7.

22. Statland JM, McDermott MP, Heatwole C, Martens WB, Pandya S, van der Kooi EL, Kissel JT, Wagner KR, Tawil R. Reevaluating measures of disease progression in facioscapulohumeral muscular dystrophy. Neuromuscul Disord. 2013;23(4):306–12.

23. Miura K, Kumagai T, Matsumoto A, Iriyama E, Watanabe K, Goto K, Arahata K. Two cases of chromosome 4q35-linked early onset facioscapulohumeral muscular dystrophy with mental retardation and epilepsy. Neuropediatrics. 1998;29(5):239–41.

24. Wijmenga C, Hewitt JE, Sandkuijl LA, Clark LN, Wright TJ, Dauwerse HG, Gruter AM, Hofker MH, Moerer P, Williamson R, et al. Chromosome 4q DNA rearrangements associated with facioscapulohumeral muscular dystrophy. Nat Genet. 1992;2(1):26–30.

25. van Deutekom JC, Wijmenga C, van Tienhoven EA, Gruter AM, Hewitt JE, Padberg GW, van Ommen GJ, Hofker MH, Frants RR. FSHD associated DNA rearrangements are due to deletions of integral copies of a 3.2 kb tandemly repeated unit. Hum Mol Genet. 1993;2(12):2037–42.

26. Hewitt JE, Lyle R, Clark LN, Valleley EM, Wright TJ, Wijmenga C, van Deutekom JC, Francis F, Sharpe PT, Hofker M, et al. Analysis of the tandem repeat locus D4Z4 associated with facioscapulohumeral muscular dystrophy. Hum Mol Genet. 1994;3(8):1287–95.

27. Wang ZQ, Wang N, van der Maarel S, Murong SX, Wu ZY. Distinguishing the 4qA and 4qB variants is essential for the diagnosis of facioscapulohumeral muscular dystrophy in the Chinese population. Eur J Hum Genet. 2011;19(1):64–9.

28. Tawil R, Kissel JT, Heatwole C, Pandya S, Gronseth G, Benatar M. Evidence-based guideline summary: Evaluation, diagnosis, and management of facioscapulohumeral musculardystrophy: Report of the Guideline Development, Dissemination, and Implementation Subcommittee of the American Academy of Neurology and the Practice Issues Review Panel of the American Association of Neuromuscular & Electrodiagnostic Medicine. Neurology. 2015;85(4):357–64.

29. Lemmers RJ, van der Vliet PJ, Klooster R, Sacconi S, Dauwerse JG, Snider L, Straasheijm KR, van Ommen GJ, Padberg GW, Miller DG, Tapscott SJ, Tawil R, Frants RR, van der Maarel SM. A unifying genetic model for facioscapulohumeral muscular dystrophy. Science. 2010;329(5999):1650–3.

30. Wallace LM, Garwick SE, Mei W, Belayew A, Coppee F, Ladner KJ, Guttridge D, Yang J, Harper SQ. DUX4, a candidate gene for facioscapulohumeral muscular dystrophy, causes p53-dependent myopathy in vivo. Ann Neurol. 2011;69(3):540–52.

31. Rickard AM, Petek LM, Miller DG. Endogenous DUX4 expression in FSHD myotubes is sufficient to cause cell death and disrupts RNA splicing and cell migration pathways. Hum Mol Genet. 2015;24(20): 5901–14.

32. Lemmers RJ, Tawil R, Petek LM, Balog J, Block GJ, Santen GW, Amell AM, van der Vliet PJ, Almomani R, Straasheijm KR, Krom YD, Klooster R, Sun Y, den Dunnen JT, Helmer Q, Donlin-Smith CM, Padberg GW, van Engelen BG, de Greef JC, Aartsma-Rus AM, Frants RR, de Visser M, Desnuelle C, Sacconi S, Filippova GN, Bakker B, Bamshad MJ, Tapscott SJ, Miller DG, van der Maarel SM. Digenic inheritance of an SMCHD1 mutation and an FSHD-permissive D4Z4 allele causes facioscapulohumeral muscular dystrophy type 2. Nat Genet. 2012;44(12):1370–4.

33. Meola G, Cardani R. Myotonic dystrophies: an update on clinical aspects, genetic, pathology, and molecular pathomechanisms. Biochim Biophys Acta. 2015; 1852(4):594–606.

34. Arsenault ME, Prévost C, Lescault A, Laberge C, Puymirat J, Mathieu J. Clinical characteristics of myotonic dystrophy type 1 patients with small CTG expansions. Neurology. 2006;66(8):1248–50.

35. Udd B, Krahe R. The myotonic dystrophies: molecular, clinical, and therapeutic challenges. Lancet Neurol. 2012;11(10):891–905.

36. Modoni A, Silvestri G, Pomponi MG, Mangiola F, Tonali PA, Marra C. Characterization of the pattern of cognitive impairment in myotonic dystrophy type 1. Arch Neurol. 2004;61(12):1943–7.

37. Schneider-Gold C, Bellenberg B, Prehn C, Krogias C, Schneider R, Klein J, Gold R, Lukas C. Cortical and subcortical grey and white matter atrophy in myotonic dystrophies type 1 and 2 is associated with cognitive impairment, depression anddaytime sleepiness. PLoS One. 2015;10(6):e0130352.

38. Minnerop M, Weber B, Schoene-Bake JC, Roeske S, Mirbach S, Anspach C, Schneider-Gold C, Betz RC, Helmstaedter C, Tittgemeyer M, Klockgether T, Kornblum C. The brain in myotonic dystrophy 1 and 2: evidence for a predominant white matter disease. Brain. 2011;134(Pt 12):3530–46.

39. Fu YH, Pizzuti A, Fenwick Jr RG, King J, Rajnarayan S, Dunne PW, Dubel J, Nasser GA, Ashizawa T, de Jong P, et al. An unstable triplet repeat in a gene related to myotonic muscular dystrophy. Science. 1992;255(5049):1256–8.

40. Brook JD, McCurrach ME, Harley HG, Buckler AJ, Church D, Aburatani H, Hunter K, Stanton VP, Thirion JP, Hudson T, et al. Molecular basis of myotonic dystrophy: expansion of a trinucleotide (CTG) repeat at the 3′ end of a transcript encoding a protein kinase family member. Cell. 1992;68(4):799–808.

41. Mulders SA, van den Broek WJ, Wheeler TM, Croes HJ, van Kuik-Romeijn P, de Kimpe SJ, Furling D, Platenburg GJ, Gourdon G, Thornton CA, Wieringa B, Wansink DG. Triplet-repeat oligonucleotide-mediated reversal of RNA toxicity in myotonic dystrophy. Proc Natl Acad Sci U S A. 2009;106(33):13915–20.

42. Musova Z, Mazanec R, Krepelova A, Ehler E, Vales J, Jaklova R, Prochazka T, Koukal P, Marikova T, Kraus J, Havlovicova M, Sedlacek Z. Highly unstable sequence interruptions of the CTG repeat in the myotonic dystrophy gene. Am J Med Genet A. 2009;149A(7):1365–74.

43. Liquori CL, Ricker K, Moseley ML, Jacobsen JF, Kress W, Naylor SL, Day JW, Ranum LP. Myotonic dystrophy type 2 caused by a CCTG expansion in intron 1 of ZNF9. Science. 2001;293(5531):864–7.

44. Kamsteeg EJ, Kress W, Catalli C, Hertz JM, Witsch-Baumgartner M, Buckley MF, van Engelen BG, Schwartz M, Scheffer H. Best practice guidelines and recommendations on the molecular diagnosis of myotonic dystrophy types 1 and 2. Eur J Hum Genet. 2012;20(12):1203–8.

45. Logigian EL, Martens WB, Moxley 4th RT, McDermott MP, Dilek N, Wiegner AW, Pearson AT, Barbieri CA, Annis CL, Thornton CA, Moxley 3rd RT. Mexiletine is an effective antimyotonia treatment in myotonic dystrophy type 1. Neurology. 2010;74(18):1441–8.

Hong-Lei Li, Yan-Bin Zhang, Sheng Chen, Bin Cai, Zhi-Jun Liu, Yan-Fang Niu, and Hao Yu

Abstract

Dementia is a broad category of neurodegenerative diseases that cause a decline in memory, the ability to acquiring knowledge and understanding that ultimately affect a person's daily functioning. Other common symptoms include a decrease in the ability of attention, judgment, problem solving, comprehension, and production of language. Psychiatric problems are also very common in patients with dementia. Dementia is often sporadic, and the prevalence is associated with aging. The most common types of dementia are Alzheimer's disease, vascular cognitive impairment, Lewy body dementia, and frontotemporal lobe degeneration. However, some hereditary disease such as Huntington's disease (HD), cerebral autosomal dominant arteriopathy with subcortical infarcts and leukoencephalopathy (CADASIL), Niemann–Pick disease (NPD), fatal familial insomnia (FFI), adrenoleukodystrophy (ALD), etc. can also manifest as cognitive impairment. However, most of these disorders present with characteristic symptoms other than cognitive decline. In this chapter, we presented several disorders with dementia or psychiatric problems caused by genetic mutations.

Keywords

Dementia • Huntington's disease • Niemann–Pick disease • Fatal familial insomnia • Adrenoleukodystrophy

H.-L. Li (✉) • Y.-B. Zhang • S. Chen • Z.-J. Liu
H. Yu
Department of Neurology and Research Center of
Neurology, Second Affiliated Hospital, Zhejiang
University School of Medicine, Hangzhou, China
e-mail: honglei2015@foxmail.com

B. Cai • Y.-F. Niu
Department of Neurology and Institute of Neurology,
First Affiliated Hospital, Fujian Medical University,
Fuzhou, China

© Springer Nature Singapore Pte Ltd. 2017
Z.-Y. Wu (ed.), *Inherited Neurological Disorders*, DOI 10.1007/978-981-10-4196-9_7

7.1 Huntington's Disease (HD)

A 25-Year-Old Woman with 9 Years of Marked Irritability and Insanity

Clinical Presentations

A 25-year-old woman complained of 9 years of irritability and insanity. Nine years ago, without rhyme or reason, the patient was noted of progressive irritability and verbal aggression toward neighbors and families. Four years later, she presented with various weird behaviors, including talking with herself often, running out at night frequently, and sometimes complaining that she heard others talking about her. So she was hospitalized in a native mental hospital. She was diagnosed initially with schizophrenia and prescribed antipsychotic medication alprazolam and olanzapine for 10 days. However, the treatment was ineffective, and several new symptoms appeared such as instable gait, frequent blink, and subtle shake in the limbs after she was discharged from the hospital. What's worse, she could only recognize close relatives. So she was transferred to our hospital soon. Her mother and grandma seemed to have a suspicious similar mental problem, and her mother had gone away from home and deceased (Fig. 7.1).

Neurological examinations in bad cooperation were conducted. The abnormal examinations included an unbalanced gait, bilateral symmetry hypermyotonia, hyperreflexia, positive ankle clonus, and pathological Babinski sign.

Her routine tests including liver and renal function tests, electrolytes, thyroid parameters, coagulation, and other blood biochemistry disclosed no remarkable abnormalities. Brain MRI revealed mild atrophy of the cerebral cortex, remarkable atrophy signals in the brainstem and cerebellum, and mild abnormal signals of the caudate nucleus and putamen ones (Fig. 7.2).

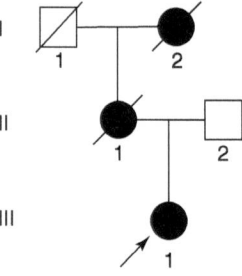

Fig. 7.1 Pedigree of the family. The patient's mother and maternal grandma seemed to have similar mental problems

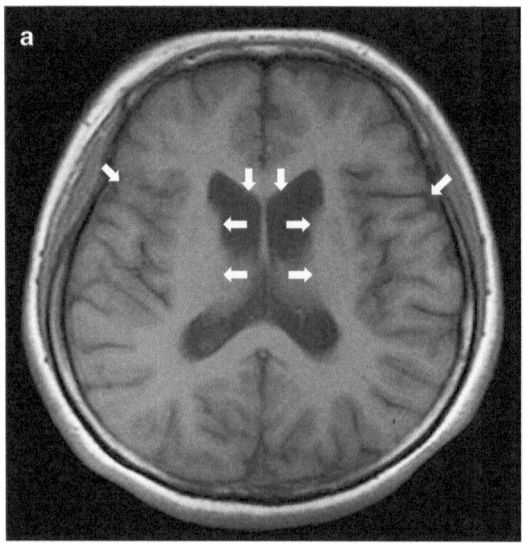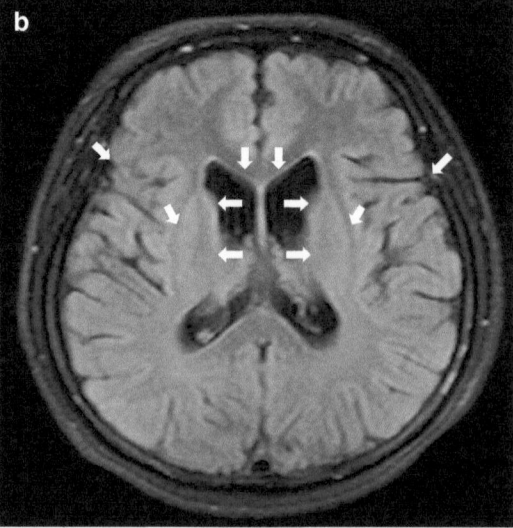

Fig. 7.2 Brain MRI (at the age of 25) showed mild atrophy signals in cerebral cortex, remarkably enlarged lateral ventricles, and atrophy signals caudate and putamen nuclei (*arrows*) of horizontal section in T1- (**a**) and T2-FLAIR (**b**)-weighted images

Primary Diagnosis

The patient's symptoms and signs indicated significant abnormal psychiatric and extrapyramidal features with rapidly exacerbated cognitive function deficit, mild ataxia, and atypical hyperkinetic. The lesions were primarily located at the cerebral cortex, basal ganglia, and cerebellum. Equivocal positive family history suggesting autosomal dominant (AD) inherited disorders should be considered. Differential diagnosis included atypical Huntington's disease (OMIM: 143,100, HD), especially juvenile HD (JHD), HD-like 4/spinocerebellar ataxia type 17 (OMIM: 607,136, HDL-4/SCA17), early onset of Parkinson's disease (OMIM: 168,600, PD) (EOPD), dentatorubral–pallidoluysian atrophy (OMIM: 125,370, DRPLA), etc. JHDs have an early onset before the age of 20 and may display rigidity, chorea, parkinsonian signs, ataxia, and schizophrenia. Although uncommon in HDL-4/SCA17, onset in childhood exists. In addition to psychiatric disturbances, HDL-4/SCA17 exhibits cerebellar ataxia, dementia, and chorea [1, 2]. DRPLA has an average age of onset between 20 and 30, and early-onset cases have clinical phenotypes of chorea, ataxia, and cognitive decline [3]. JHD, HDL-4/SCA17, and DRPLA probably have positive family history. EOPD has genetic and clinical heterogeneity which could company psychiatric disturbances and parkinsonism [4]. In order to confirm the genetic disease, accurate related gene tests must be conducted.

Additional Tests or Key Results

Since HD is the leading inherited cause of chorea with ataxia, cognitive, and psychiatric symptoms, JHD disease should be considered first on this young patient. *HUNTINGTIN* (OMIM: 613,004, *HTT*) gene (the causative gene for HD) molecular test was conducted, and abnormal trinucleotide repeats were found (Fig. 7.3a). Genetic sequencing subsequently revealed that the aberrant repeat number was 59 (Fig. 7.3b).

Discussion

HD is a relatively rare hereditary degenerative disease, especially in Chinese [5], mainly characterized by involuntary chorea, behavioral or psychiatric disorders, and progressive dementia clinically [6, 7]. It's caused by CAG repeat expansion beyond 40 within *HTT* gene [8–10], whose molecular test plays a key role in quick and specific diagnosis [11]. Most patients initiate chorea movement insidiously in 30–40s [12] and usually have positive family history.

JHD could be quite different from the typical adult HD. They present symptoms before the age of 20 years and the earliest at 18 months old [13]. Unlike representative HD, JHDs usually are manifested by the atypical presentations including behavioral, cognitive, psychiatric, and emotional symptoms, parkinsonian signs, and ataxia [14–17]. Although JHD could develop chorea as one of the first symptoms, chorea is uncommon particularly in the early stage of children with HD.

The marked mental problems in this JHD case misled relatives and psychiatrists. Delayed chorea and unremarkable walking instability, dubious family history, and no remarkable basal ganglia abnormal in brain MRI in the beginning also covered up the important hints to the fact. Above all, lack of experience about this rare hereditary disease would easily result in misdiagnosis. Accordingly, JHD should be considered in young patients suffering from abrupt psychiatric problems and neurological disorders, especially those with positive family history, no matter they had striatal atrophy in image or not.

HD is a dominantly inherited disorder with various symptoms. There is no cure so far, and pharmacological treatment attempted is aimed at symptomatic and supportive care. Tetrabenazine (TBZ) remains the only medication approved by FDA for chorea. The hunt for other effective symptom relief in HD, such as coenzyme Q10 or creatine, might have shown effectivity [17]. It's necessary to carefully review the pharmaceutical instructions before prescribing any psychiatric medication [18], such as antipsychotic risperidone and antidepressant sertraline used for depression or irritability and anxiety.

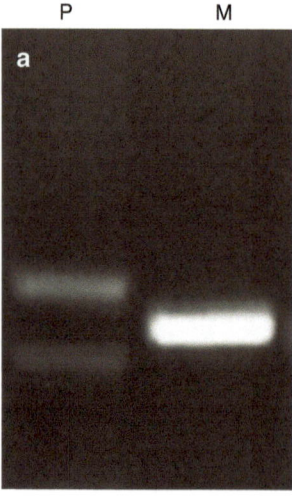

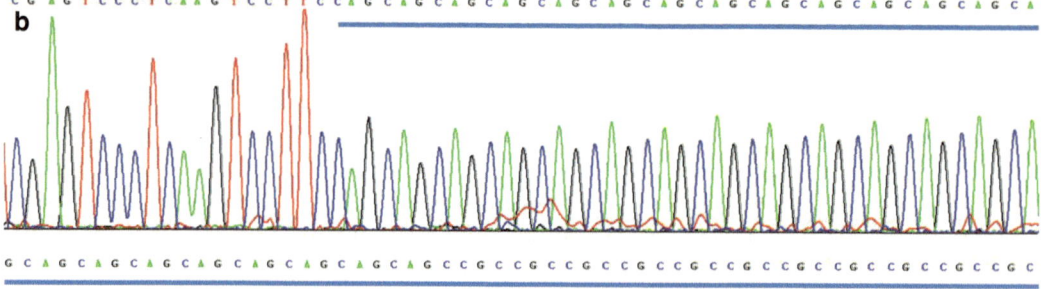

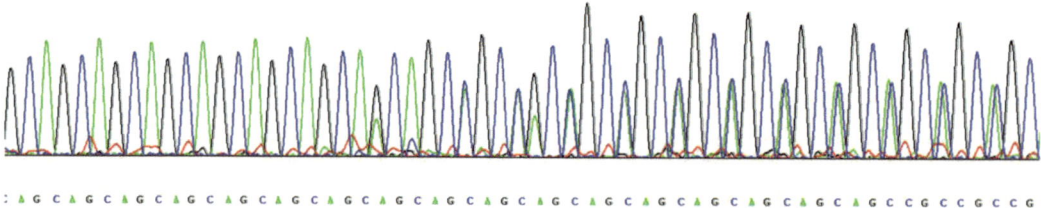

CAG repeats

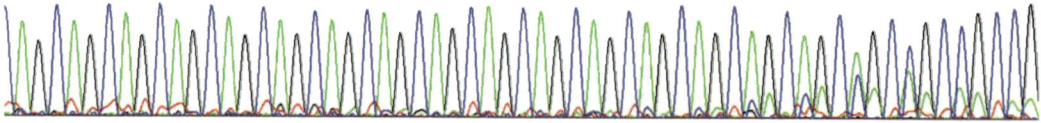

Fig. 7.3 Mutation analysis of the patient. (**a**) *P* patient, two separated bands showed different lengths of CAG repeats of *HTT* gene from both alleles; the upper one was normal and the lower one referred to expanded CAG repeats. *M* marker of 309 bp corresponding to 35 CAG repeats. (**b**) Chromatogram of *HTT* gene in the patient showed normal allele with 17 CAG repeats and expanded allele with 59 CAG repeats. The *blue arrows* indicated the abnormal CAG repeats

7.2 Cerebral Autosomal Dominant Arteriopathy with Subcortical Infarcts and Leukoencephalopathy (CADASIL)

A 44-Year-Old Man with Recurrent Headache and Memory Loss

Clinical Presentations

A 44-year-old man was referred to our neurology clinic for half a year of recurrent headache. The headache was usually located in the occipital region. When asked to describe his headache pain, the patient reported dull pain. He also reported that he experienced at least one episode per month and each headache episode usually lasted for a few hours. In addition, the patient admitted that he was becoming impatient and irritated and frequently forgot his keys. No history of hypertension, no fever, no seizures, and no limb weakness were reported. Brain MRI scanning at a local hospital revealed small ischemic foci scattering in frontal–parietal lobes and white matter hyperintensities (WMH) mainly involving bilateral periventricular areas and anterior temporal lobes (Fig. 7.4a–d). He also claimed that his father (I_1) died of stroke at 62 (Fig. 7.5a).

Primary Diagnosis

The patient's headache and memory loss were closely associated with subcortical white matter lesions in his brain. Nevertheless, the MRI images showed more lesions without any clinical presentation. The mild to moderate WMH in MRI and mood disturbance were strong reminders for cerebral small vessel diseases (SVD), such as hypertensive arteriopathy (IIA), cerebral autosomal dominant arteriopathy with subcortical infarcts and leukoencephalopathy (CADASIL), cerebral amyloid angiopathy (CAA), and so on. However, the HA should be excluded because the patient reported no history of hypertension. Besides, no

lobar hemorrhage occurred and a young age can exclude CAA. Considering his specific WMH in bilateral anterior temporal lobes as well as external capsules and his suspected autosomal dominant family history, the diagnosis of CADASIL was suspected, and a gene test for CADASIL was arranged.

Additional Tests or Key Results

He received a Wechsler Adult Intelligence Scale Revised by China (WAIS-RC), and a Wechsler Memory Scale Revised by China (WMS-RC) in our center considered a complain of memory loss. He scored 88, 104, and 95 in verbal intelligence quotient (VIQ), performance intelligence quotient (PIQ), and full intelligence quotient (FIQ), respectively. However, his score in WMS-RC was below 51. The remaining neurological examinations were unremarkable. A brain MRI scanning with fluid-attenuated inversion recovery (FLAIR) sequence was performed in the patient and revealed similar lesions compared to the former scanning at the local hospital but with more lacunar foci and severe WMH (Fig. 7.4e–h). Also, mutation analysis of *NOTCH3* revealed a c.1819C>T (p.R607C) mutation (Fig. 7.5b) in exon 11 of *NOTCH3*, which confirmed the patient's diagnosis of CADASIL.

Discussion

CADASIL is a dominant inherited cerebral arteriopathy characterized by adult-onset recurrent subcortical infarctions, cognitive decline, episodic headache, sometimes migraine, and psychiatric symptoms [19]. It is caused by mutations within *NOTCH3* gene, which encodes a single-pass transmembrane Notch3 receptor containing 34 epidermal growth factor repeats (EGFR) [20]. Mutations leading to an odd number of cysteine residues within each EGFR in extracellular domain of Notch3 might be pathogenic. To date, over 270 mutations have been reported, and the majority of them occur in exons 2–24. Though it has not been well confirmed, there are several "hot regions"

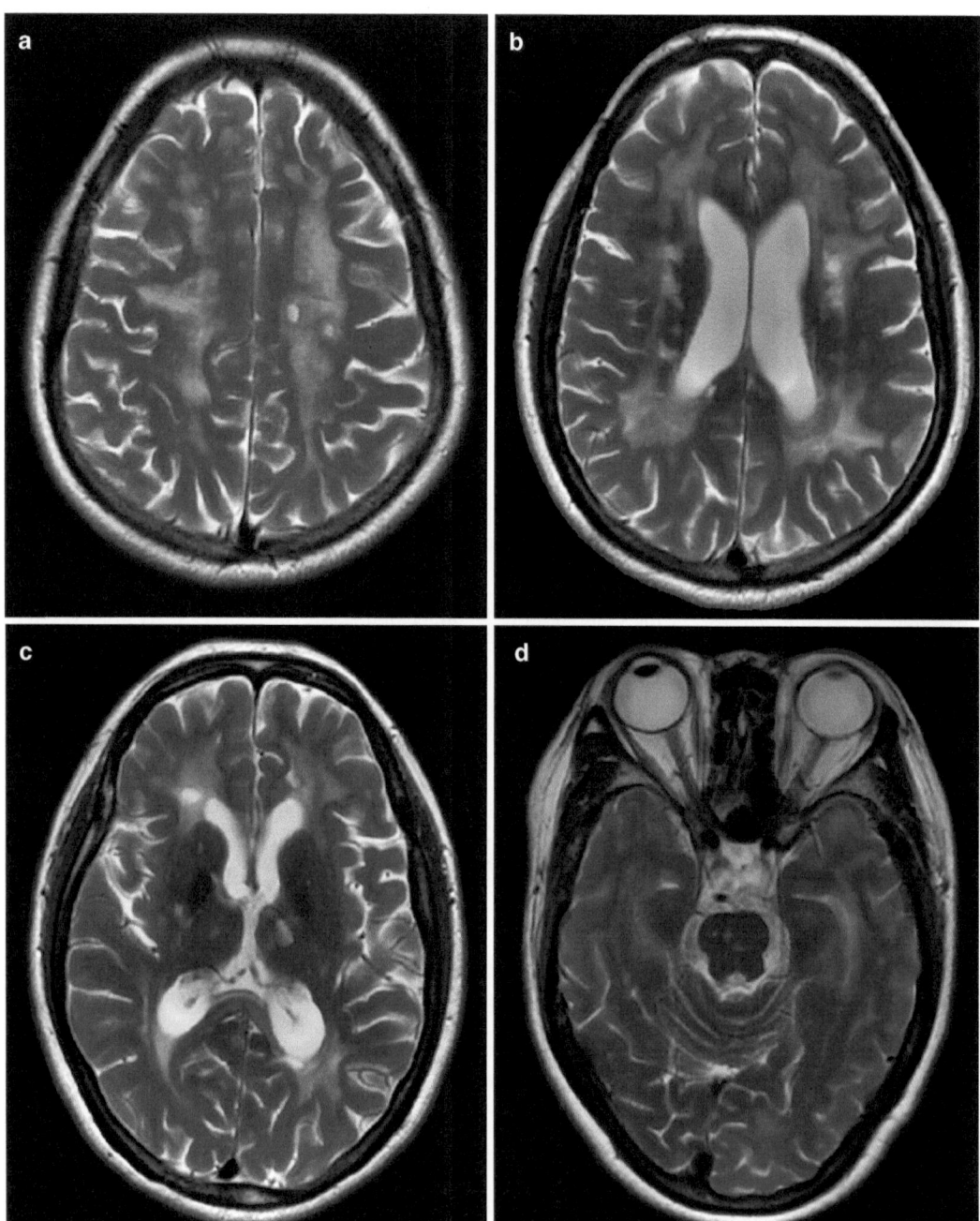

Fig. 7.4 Brain MRI of the patient. (**a**) T2-weighted axial image through the level of subcortical showing scattered small ischemic foci in frontal and parietal lobes and semi-oval center. (**b**) T2-weighted axial image through the level of lateral ventricles showing severe white matter hyperintensities (WMH) in periventricular areas. (**c**) T2-weighted axial image through the level of pineal region showing small ischemic foci in basal ganglia and right external capsule. (**d**) T2-weighted axial image through the level of sella turcica showing WMH in the brainstem and bilateral anterior temporal lobes. (**e**) Fluid-attenuated inversion recovery (FLAIR) image through the level of subcortical showing scattered small ischemic foci in frontal and parietal lobes and semioval center. (**f**) FLAIR image through the level of lateral ventricles showing severe WMH in periventricular areas. (**g**) FLAIR image through the level of pineal region showing small ischemic foci in basal ganglia and right external capsule. (**h**) FLAIR image through the level of sella turcica showing WMH in bilateral anterior temporal lobes

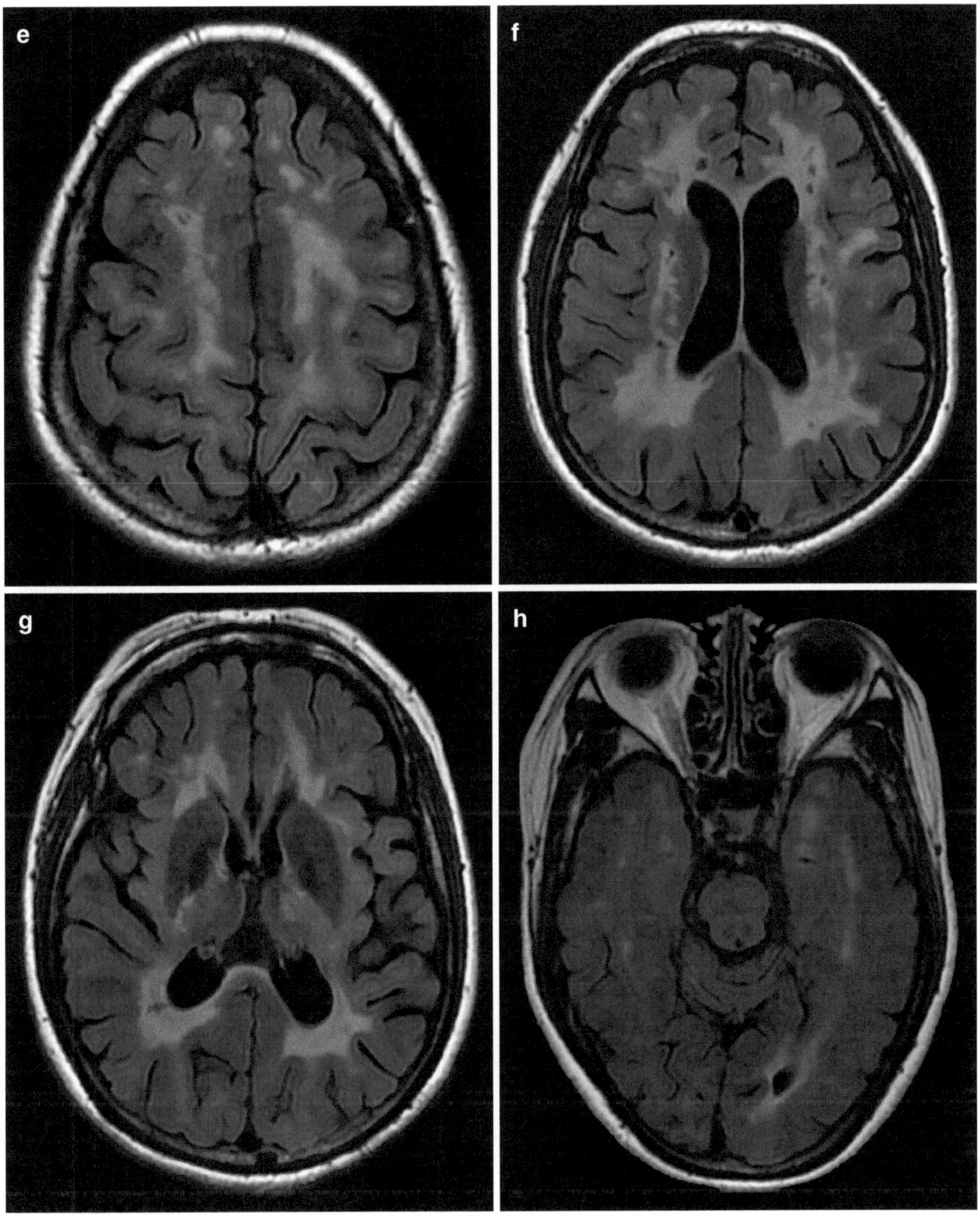

Fig. 7.4 (continued)

which have been identified. For instance, in Northern China as well as several Western countries, the exons 3 and 4 were supposed to be "hot regions" followed by exons 8, 5, 6, and 11 [21–23]. Nevertheless, the spectrum of mutations in Southern China differed. It seems that mutations located in exon 11 may be more frequent, and the mutation c.1630C>T (p.R544C) has been identified as a "hot spot" in Han Chinese in Taiwan, where it is located in Southeastern China [24]. In this case, our patient, from Shanghai, carried a previously reported mutation located in exon 11 as well.

a

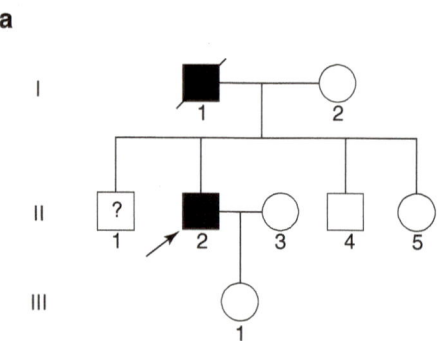

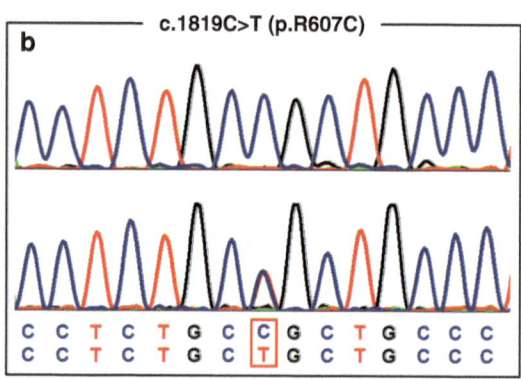

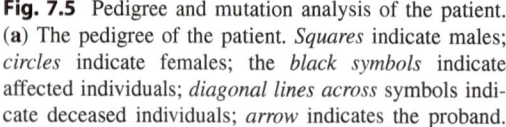

Fig. 7.5 Pedigree and mutation analysis of the patient. (a) The pedigree of the patient. *Squares* indicate males; *circles* indicate females; the *black symbols* indicate affected individuals; *diagonal lines across* symbols indicate deceased individuals; *arrow* indicates the proband.

(b) Chromatogram of c.1819C>T (p.R607C) mutation in *NOTCH3*. The *upper panel* represents heterozygous mutated sequence of the patient, whereas the *lower panel* is normal sequence of the control

Patients who suffered from CADASIL may present a variety of clinical manifestations. However, the incidence rate of each symptom varies among populations. Migraine with aura has been reported to be presented in 20–40% of the CADASIL patients in Caucasian populations [25]. Nevertheless, the occurrence in Han Chinese in Southeastern China might not be beyond 1.8% based on a recent research [24], which means less migraine might be presented in Southeastern China. In our case, the patient complained of headache but not migraine as well.

The MRI features are usually key clues for diagnosis of CADASIL. Like which in our case, the MRI changes of CADASIL patients are often characterized as white matter involvement in bilateral external capsules and anterior temporal lobes, as well as lacunar infarcts. Once these MRI features are identified, mutation analysis of

NOTCH3 or a skin biopsy should be highly recommended. It has been reported that the deposits of granular osmiophilic material (GOM) in the basal layer of vascular smooth muscle cells (VSMCs) were considered the most common pathognomonic feature of CADASIL [26]. However, the sensitivity of skin biopsies varied from 44% to nearly 100% [26, 27]. It is supposed that the detection of GOM requires more technically accuracy, whereas the gene test is showing its convenience in the diagnosis of CADASIL.

Since the patient was diagnosed as CADASIL, he was then prescribed with cilostazol. Aspirin and clopidogrel should be avoided. Once if the patient presented cardiovascular risk factors, such as hypertension, diabetes, or hyperlipidemia, corresponding treatments should be more active. The cigarette and alcohol consumptions should be prevented as well.

7.3 Cerebral Autosomal Recessive Arteriopathy with Subcortical Infarcts and Leukoencephalopathy (CARASIL)[1]

A 28-Year-Old Man with Limb Weakness and Alopecia

Clinical Presentations

The proband, a 28-year-old male, was admitted to a local hospital because of sudden lower limb weakness and thigh numbness for 2 months, the brain MRI revealed multiple abnormal signals, and the patient was diagnosed with multiple sclerosis (MS) and treated with 500 mg methylprednisolone for 5 days. He experienced hair loss, starting 10 years prior, which developed into alopecia (Fig. 7.6). The patient experienced low back pain and was diagnosed with a lumbar herniated disc by CT scan. No hypertension, diabetes mellitus, or dyslipidemia was recorded. He had no history of cigarette smoking or alcohol use. His parents had a consanguineous marriage

(Fig. 7.7), and their neuroimaging examination was normal.

Neurological examinations on the proband revealed mood and personality changes, slurred speech, muscle strength of proximal right lower limb of 5 level, and left of 3 level, respectively. Diffuse pyramidal signs, including muscle stiffness, increased tendon reflexes, left ankle clonus, and bilateral Babinski signs. Sensation to pain and light touch in both lower extremities diminished. Mini-Mental State Examination (MMSE) was normal.

A follow-up MRI showed diffuse leukoencephalopathy, subcortical infarcts, and microbleeds (Fig. 7.8). Visual evoked potentials (VEP)

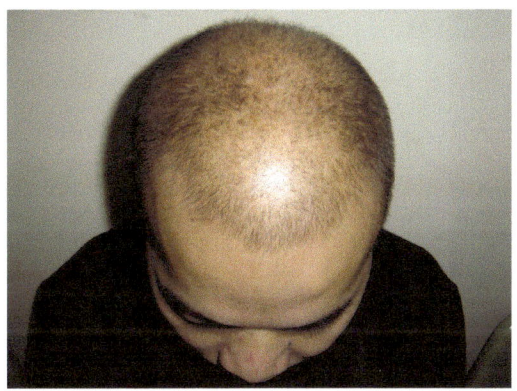

Fig. 7.6 The proband developed alopecia with male pattern baldness

---

[1] This section is reprinted with permission from: Cai B, Zeng JB, Lin Y, et al. (2015) A frameshift mutation in HTRA1 expands CARASIL syndrome and peripheral small arterial disease to the Chinese population. NeurolSci 36(8):1387–91.

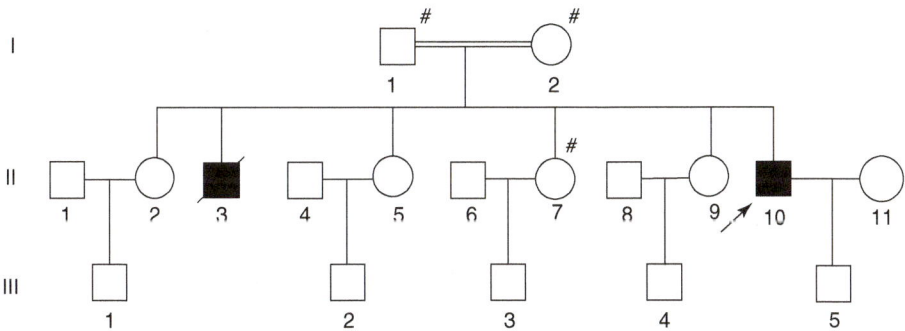

Fig. 7.7 The pedigree of family with CARASIL. The proband is indicated by the *arrow*. The *solid symbols* denote the patient with CARASIL, and the symbol with a *slash* indicates the deceased individual. *Double horizontal lines*: consanguineous marriage; *hash*, unaffected individuals with a heterozygous c.161_162insAG mutation

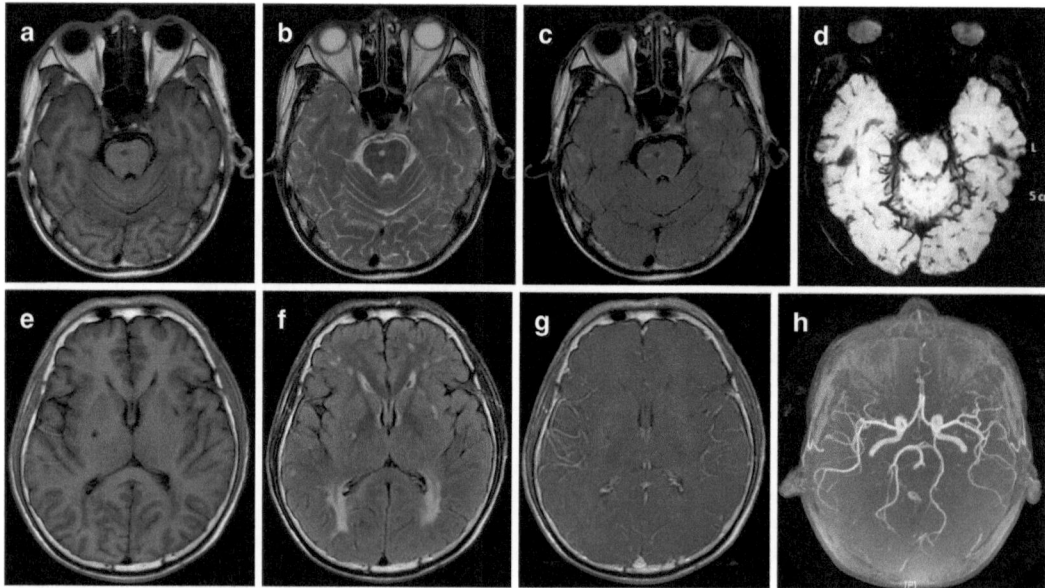

Fig. 7.8 Brain MRI of the proband. T1 weighted (**a**, **e**), T2 weighted (**b**, **f**), and fluid-attenuated inversion recovery (FLAIR). (**c**) MRI showed diffuse leukoencephalopathy involving the periventricular and deep white matter, including the anterior temporal lobes and external capsules, and multiple lacunar infarcts in the brain hemispheres and brainstem. No significant strengthening of

enhanced lesions (**g**); susceptibility-weighted image (SWI) (**d**) of MRI showed multiple cerebral microbleeds (CMBs) on the pons, basal ganglia, and hemispheric subcortical white matter. A brain magnetic resonance angiogram (MRA) showed no significant stenosis of large cerebral arteries (**h**)

were normal, oligoclonal bands in CSF were absent, and ultrasonic doppler showed bilateral vertebral arteries supplying a high-resistance vascular bed. Transcranial doppler (TCD) indicated increased cerebrovascular resistance. Single-photon emission computed tomography (SPECT) revealed reduced perfusion in the left frontotemporal lobe.

The proband's older brother was admitted to our department because of a similar neurological history (Fig. 7.7) in 2002, when he was 29 years old. He also developed alopecia and a lumbar herniated disc. The neurological examinations and MRI results were similar to the proband, and he was diagnosed with MS and treated with prednisolone. However, pseudobulbar syndrome and tetraparesis progressed until he was bedridden at age 30 and died at age 32.

Primary Diagnosis

The symptoms and signs of this patient hint the involvement of pyramid sign, sensation disorder, a slurred speech, respectively, mood and per-

sonality changes, and worsening problems with movement. Taken together, these disclose the extensive impairment of the central nervous system (CNS).

The differential diagnosis includes MS and cerebral small vessel diseases (CSVDs) caused by cerebral autosomal dominant arteriopathy with subcortical infarcts and leukoencephalopathy (CADASIL) or other reasons. VEP and lumbar puncture were normal, which disagreed the diagnosis of MS and immunity diseases.

Diffuse leukoencephalopathy, subcortical infarcts, and microbleeds in MRI supported the diagnosis of CSVDs. The hypothesis of CADASIL was first considered, so the *NOTCH3* gene analysis from the blood should be performed to exclude this diagnosis. Other characteristic features of these brothers include premature hair loss (alopecia) and attacks of low back pain, which are characteristic extraneurological signs of cerebral autosomal recessive arteriopathy with subcortical infarcts and leukoencephalopathy (CARASIL), suggesting the diagnosis of CARASIL. Thus,

HTRA1 gene analysis from the blood should be performed to confirm the diagnosis.

Additional Tests or Key Results

No *NOTCH3* mutation in the blood and ultrastructural granular osmiophilic material (GOM) on the vascular wall was found, which excluded the diagnosis of CADASIL. Spine MRI showed degenerative disc disease (Fig. 7.9), and a novel homozygous frameshift mutation (c.161_162insAG) within *HTRA1* gene, leading to the formation of a stop codon 159 amino acids downstream of the insertion (p.Gly56Alafs*160), was detected in the proband (Fig. 7.10), which confirmed the diagnosis of CARASIL.

Discussion

CARASIL is a rare single-gene disorder directly affecting the cerebral small vessels; is characterized by nonhypertensive cerebral small-vessel arteriopathy with subcortical infarcts, alopecia, and low back pain; and has an onset in early adulthood [28, 29]. The first CARASIL patients were most likely described in preliminary reports in 1965, and approximately 50

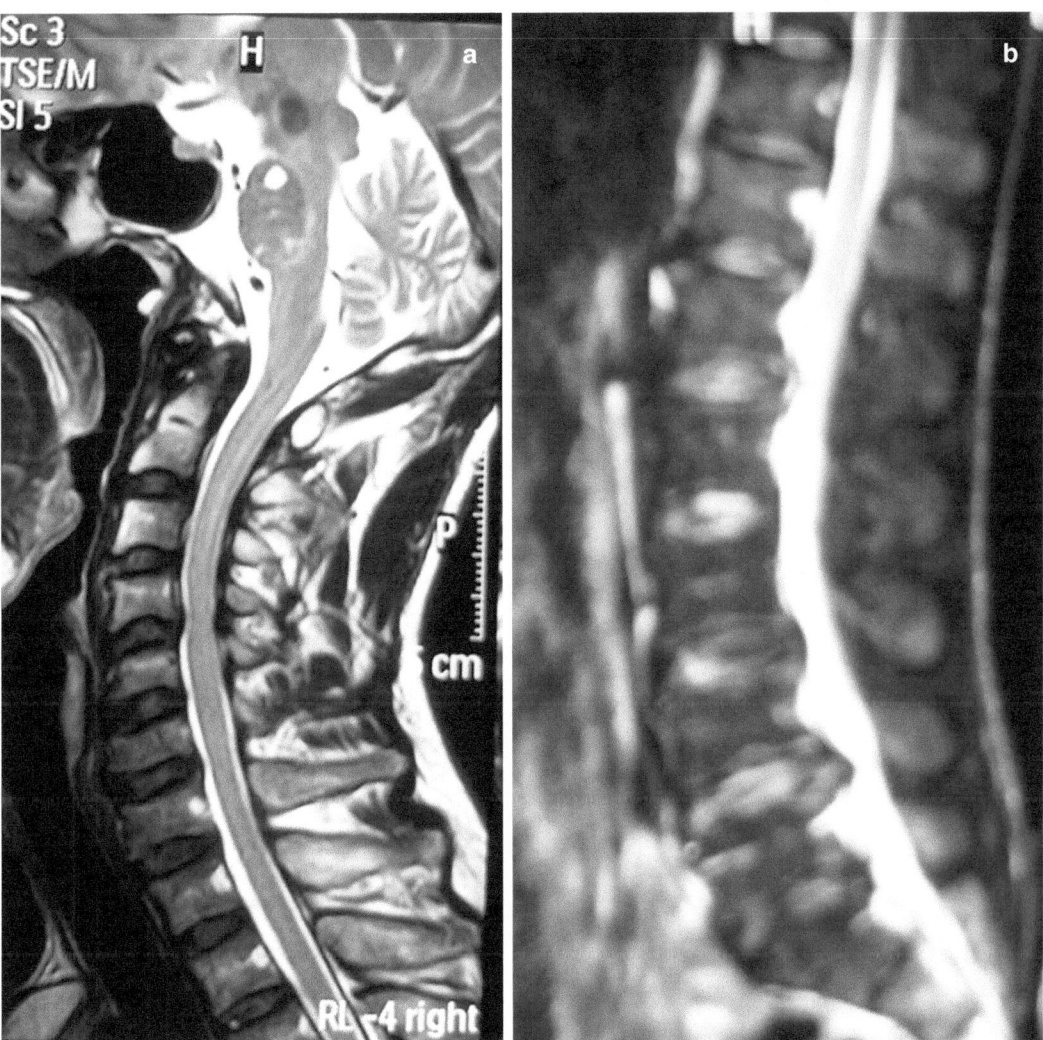

Fig. 7.9 Cervical and lumbar spine MRI of the proband. T2-weighted images show degenerative disc disease, including disc herniations and the degeneration of vertebral bodies

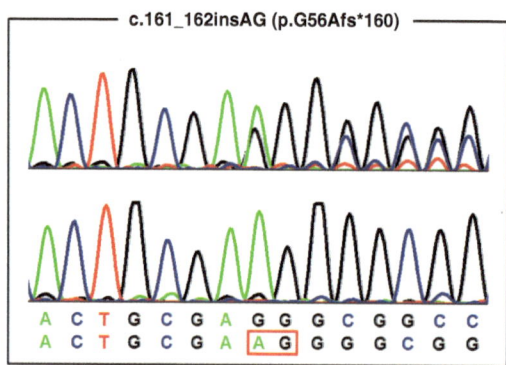

c.161_162insAG (p.G56Afs*160)

A C T G C G A G G G C G G C C
A C T G C G A [A G] G G G C G G

Fig. 7.10 Mutation analysis of *HTRA1* in the proband identified a novel homozygous mutation (c.161_162insAG)

patients, primarily from Japan, have been reported; more patients are also being reported in other populations [30–33]. In 2009, the HtrA serine protease 1 gene (*HTRA1*) was identified by Hara et al. [34] as the causative gene of CARASIL. *HTRA1* is located on chromosome 10 and encodes an enzyme that regulates signaling by the TGF-β family of proteins. TGF-β plays an important role in cellular functions, specifically angiogenesis.

The proband and his brother were misdiagnosed and initially treated as MS because of cerebral white matter lesions on brain MRI. Nonetheless, the diagnosis of CARASIL was confirmed by a novel homozygous mutation in exon 1 (c.161_162insAG) of the *HTRA1* gene detected in the proband. The deleterious effect of this mutation is supported by the following arguments.

Firstly, the mutation in exon 1 (c.161_162insAG) of the *HTRA1* gene leads to a frameshift that results in the formation of a stop codon 159 amino acids downstream of the insertion (p.Gly56Alafs*160) and produces a truncated protein without the proteolytic (trypsin-like) and PDZ domains. As the serine protease activity of *HTRA1* is required to inhibit TGF-β family

signaling, the loss of *HTRA1* protein caused by the mutation will result in the failure to repress signaling by the TGF-β family, which increases TGF-β1 expression. TGF-β family signaling is associated with vascular angiogenesis and remodeling; thus, the increased TGF-β1 expression will result in cerebral small vessel diseases.

Secondly, ultrasonic doppler and TCD showed increased cerebrovascular resistance, and SPECT showed reduced cerebral blood flow; all of these tests suggested the stenosis of cerebral small arteries. Arteriosclerosis observed in cerebral small arteries, including the hyaline degeneration of the media, loss of vascular SMCs, and the thickening and splitting of the internal elastic lamina [31], is a characteristic feature of CARASIL [35]. Arteriosclerosis was also reported in the peripheral small arteries in other organs but not in the skin. Peripheral small arterial disease including the loss of vascular SMCs and thickening and splitting of the internal elastic lamina was found in the subcutaneous tissue, which was consistent with the results reported previously [30, 36].

Thirdly, we detected decreased *HTRA1* and increased TGF-β1 protein expression [31] in the subcutaneous tissue and cultured fibroblasts by western blot and IHC [37], which may be attributable to the *HTRA1* mutation. The small arterial disease in the subcutaneous tissue may be caused by the mutation in *HTRA1* because this protein is expressed in the skin as well as in the brain [28].

The diagnosis of CARASIL should be considered in patients with previously suspected atypical MS, CADASIL, especially in patients with the extraneurological signs, including scalp alopecia in the teens and acute mid to lower back pain. The diagnosis can be confirmed by *HTRA1* genetic testing.

7.4 Adrenoleukodystrophy (ALD)

A 12-Year-Old Boy with Impairment of Cognition, Deafness, and Blindness

Clinical Presentations

A 12-year-old boy suffered from rapidly progressive impairment of cognition 1 year ago, unstable gait, and visual and auditory impairment 3 months ago. One week ago he exhibited dysphagia and slurred speech. He presented with a decline of school performance at the beginning. His cognition was progressively impaired during the last 1 year, and he had learning deficits and could not remember familiar situation. He experienced weakness of both lower limbs with difficulty climbing stairs. From 2 months ago, his emotionality changed, he easily cries or laughs, and he was becoming deaf and blind. He had swallowing problem and slurred speech 1 week ago. Medical history revealed unremarkable birth and growth milestones except for a history of chicken pox at 9 years old.

Neurological examinations revealed slurred speech and dementia. The patient also exhibited left ipsilateral visual field defect and left central facial and lingual paralysis. He presented stagger gait. His muscle strength was 3–4/5 (MRCS, grades 0–5). Both lower limbs and left arm were spastic. His deep tendon reflex was hyperactive with 3+ at biceps, triceps, and radial periosteal, 4+ at the knees and Achilles. Bilateral ankle clonus and Babinski sign were positive in this patient. Left upper and lower extremities were dysmetria. His sensory examinations were symmetric.

Electrocardiography, chest radiography, and upper abdominal and kidney ultrasonography disclosed unremarkable findings. The blood routine examinations also disclosed unremarkable findings. Laboratory data showed the level of blood cortisol, and adrenocorticotropic hormone was normal. Generalized cerebral atrophy was seen on magnetic resonance imaging (MRI) of the brain. Brain MRI showed confluent and symmetric hyperintensities involving triangular area of bilateral cerebral ventricle on T2-FLAIR sequences (Fig. 7.11).

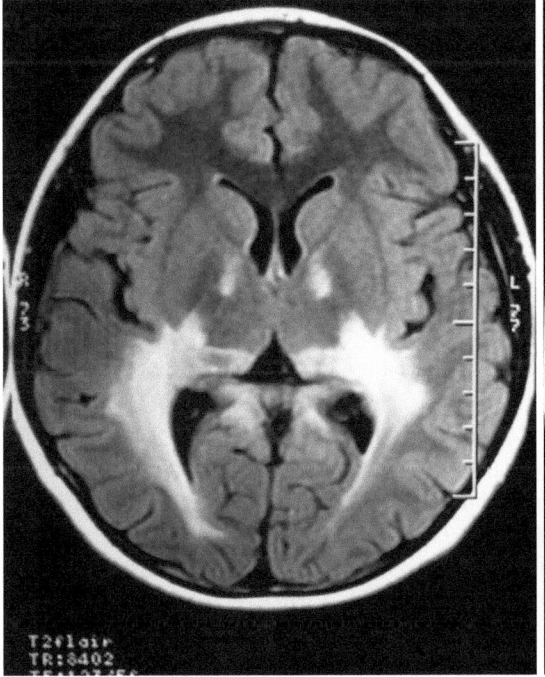 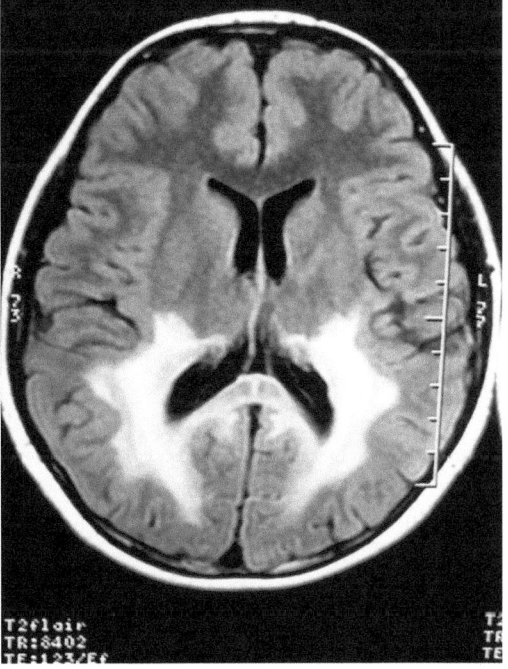

Fig. 7.11 Brain MRI of the patient. T2-FLAIR image through the level of basal ganglia showing confluent and symmetric white matter hyperintensities in triangular area of bilateral cerebral ventricle. Focal white matter lesion in the splenium of the corpus callosum is the symmetric butterfly shape

Primary Diagnosis

The symptoms and signs of this patient including the involvement of cognition, visual field defect, unstable gait, trouble in swallowing, and slurred speech indicating that the lesions were bilaterally cortex, brainstem, cone bundle, and cerebellum, respectively. Taken together, these disclose the extensive impairment of central nervous system.

The long progressive course of disease and brain MRI implied that hereditary metabolic diseases such as X-linked adrenoleukodystrophy (ALD) should be considered first for this patient. The differential diagnosis includes infectious diseases, multiple sclerosis, mitochondrial encephalomyopathy, hereditary spastic paraparesis with amyotrophy, metachromatic leukodystrophy, and Krabbe disease.

Lumbar puncture is necessary to exclude the infection and immunity disease. Organic acid test from the blood and urine is needed to verify some metabolic disorders (such as deficiencies of vitamin B12, folic acid, copper). Also, molecular analysis of *ABCD1* gene is necessary.

Additional Tests or Key Results

Lumbar puncture showed normal results. Plasma concentration of very-long-chain fatty acids (VLCFA) was normal. The concentration of C26:0 and the ratio of C24:0/C22:0 and C26:0/C22:0 were normal. The sequencing of *ABCD1* gene revealed that the patient harbored ABCD1 c.1661G>A mutation, which resulted in the protein substitution of p.R554H (Fig. 7.12). The further sequencing revealed the patient's mother and brother didn't carry this mutation.

Discussion

From the history, neuroimaging, and molecular genetic testing, we can diagnose the boy with X-ALD, which is the most common leukodystrophy with an estimated incidence of 1 in 17,000 newborns (males and females combined) [38]. It is a progressive, neurometabolic disease that affects the brain, spinal cord, peripheral nerves, adrenal cortex, and testis. The disease is caused by mutations in the *ABCD1* gene, located at chromosome Xq28, which encodes for the peroxisomal membrane protein participating in the transmembrane

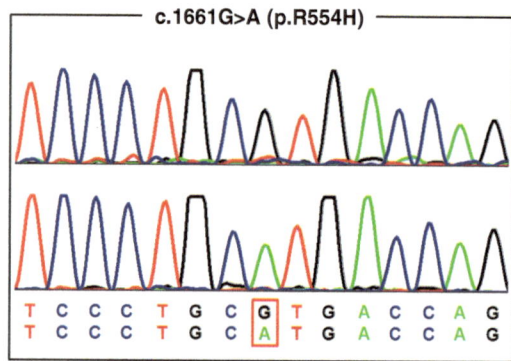

Fig. 7.12 Mutation analysis of the patient. Chromatogram of c.1661G>A (p.R554H) mutation in *ABCD1*. The *upper panel* represents normal sequence of the control, whereas the *lower panel* is mutated sequence of the patient

transport of VLCFA (≥C22) [39–41]. A defect in the ABCD1 protein results in elevated concentrations of VLCFA in plasma and tissues.

X-ALD is described as an inherited disease with wide different phenotypes. The phenotypes can be subdivided into four main categories: cerebral ALD, AMN (adrenomyeloneuropathy), Addison only, and asymptomatic. Cerebral ALD is the most rapidly progressive and devastating phenotype. Cerebral ALD occurs often in childhood (childhood cerebral ALD; CCALD) [42]. Usually, affected children initially have attention deficits or hyperactivity and then followed by progressive behavioral disturbance, vision loss, worsening handwriting, incoordination, and so on. Progressive impairment of brain often leads to total disability within 2 years. Brain MRI often provides the first lead to the diagnosis of X-ALD. In approximately 85% of patients with X-ALD, brain MRI shows a classic pattern of symmetrical enhanced T-2 signal in the parieto-occipital region, and the advancing margin is contrast enhanced [43]. The plasma level of VLCFA is abnormal in 99% of affected individuals [39, 44]. *ABCD1* is the only gene known to be associated with ALD. Over 700 different mutations have been identified in *ABCD1*. All proven pathogenic mutations identified in the *ABCD1* gene are catalogued on X-ALD database (http://www.x-ald.nl). Many ALD kindreds have a unique mutation.

Diagnosis of X-ALD is based on the clinical features, increased concentration of VLCFA, and the genetic evidence of the *ABCD1* mutations. For this patient, his age of onset is about 10 years old, and he has a rapidly progressive duration. He performed deficits in cognitive abilities at the beginning. This early clinical symptoms are often misdiagnosed as attention deficit hyperactivity disorder. As the disease progresses, more obvious neurologic deficits became apparent, which include auditory impairment, decreased visual acuity, spastic tetraparesis, and cerebellar ataxia. His brain MRI shows a typical symmetrical enhanced T-2 signal in the parieto-occipital region. Mutation analysis of *ABCD1* identified a proved pathogenic mutation (c.1661G>A). However, the patient's mother and brother didn't have this mutation. It has been reported that about 93% of index cases have inherited the *ABCD1* mutation from the mother, while 7% of cases have de novo mutations [44].

Treatment for ALD is a major challenge. When adrenal insufficiency is identified in an affected patient, corticosteroid replacement therapy is essential and can be lifesaving, but have no effect on damage inflicted to the nervous system. A lipid diet with restricted intake of very-long-chain fatty acids has proved effective in normalizing the level of very-long-chain fatty acids in plasma, but does not appear to alter the course of neurologic progression in patients who already have neurologic symptoms [45].

7.5   Fatal Familial Insomnia (FFI)

A 59-Year-Old Man with Psychiatric Abnormality and Progressive Memory Loss

Clinical Presentations

A 59-year-old man was admitted with a complaint of psychiatric abnormality coupled with progressive memory loss for a period of 4 months. He developed psychiatric abnormality, characterized by visual hallucination and mild paranoia 4 months ago. And he also exhibited obvious cognitive decline, poor disorientation, as well as personality change at that time. Soon after these symptoms, he has trouble falling asleep and even sometimes experienced insomnia throughout the whole night. Two months later, he developed involuntary grasping movements and had too much nonsense speech while asleep, which would disappear after being woken up. He also had severe walking instability, mild dysphagia, and frequent occurrence of upper and lower extremity myoclonus. Then he was admitted to a local psychiatric hospital and diagnosed with organic mental disorders. He was discharged soon from the hospital after receiving a few days treatment with sodium valproate and vitamins, but didn't get any significant improvement in his symptoms.

Nothing else of note was found in his past medical history. He had a history of more than 20 years of alcohol dependence with approximate 200 mL of white wine per day. In his family, his father experienced similar symptoms in his 40s (Fig. 7.13) and passed away 6 months after symptom onset. Since the beginning of the disease, the patient was in a bad mental state. He underwent a severe trouble of sleep disturbance, frequent constipation, and a kilogram weight loss in the past 4 months.

On neurological examination, he was apathetic. He had severe impairment in calculating, orientation, as well as the short-term memory. Examination of cranial nerves revealed unremarkable signs except for the reduced gag reflex. Deep tendon reflexes were hyperactive symmetrically. Muscle tone was obviously increased. Pathological signs were bilaterally positive. The spontaneous myoclonus of the upper and lower extremity was also observed. In terms of coordination ability, finger–nose testing was positive, but heel-to-shin testing was normal. Gait testing revealed imbalance on standing. His sensory examinations were normal.

Laboratory tests revealed the following abnormalities: ALT of 87U/L, AST of 47U/L, LDH of 217U/L, pre-meal blood glucose level of 8.1 mmol/L, serum progesterone level of <0.64 nmol/L, and vit B12 level of 1116 pmol/L. Routine cytological and biochemical examination of CSF disclosed unremarkable findings. The CSF total protein (67.2 mg/dL) was slightly increased. The brain MRI revealed mild cortical atrophic changes. EEG revealed intermittent appearance of diffuse α-wave and θ-waves in bilateral cerebral hemispheres.

During the 14 hospitalization days, he was treated with Aricept, Sinemet, clozapine, clonazepam, and other neurotropic drugs to alleviate his symptoms. His mental state was significantly ameliorated, but the sleep problem wasn't improved. Telephone follow-up in the second month after discharge we were told that the patient's condition deteriorated rapidly and had passed away 7 months after symptom onset.

Primary Diagnosis

In general, the patient presented with a midlife onset and short clinical course. The severe psychiatric symptoms, obvious cognitive decline, and apathy could be explained by lesions of cerebral cortex. The involuntary grasping movements and spontaneous myoclonus also suggested the impairment of cerebral cortex. Neurological examinations revealed the involvement of the pyramidal system. Level diagnosis was thus located at the cerebral cortex, and pyramidal system. In addition, constipation was

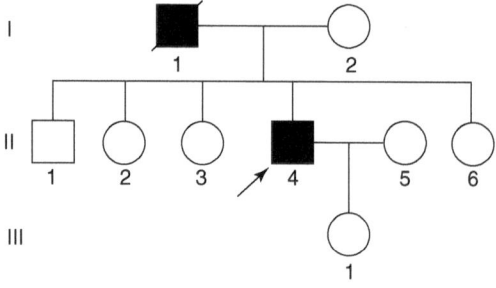

Fig. 7.13 The pedigree of the patient. *Squares* indicate males; *circles* indicate females; the *black symbols* indicate affected individuals; *diagonal lines across* symbols indicate deceased individuals; *arrow* indicates the proband

the direct evidence of autonomic disturbances. Elevated sugar levels and decreased progesterone levels were manifestations of endocrine disorder. Taken together, multiple systems of the body were involved in the disease. Based on the typical feature of acute midlife onset and rapid progressive dementia in present case, the possible etiologies were infection and inflammation. The main differential diagnosis included Creutzfeldt–Jakob disease, encephalitis, autoimmune encephalopathies, and dementia with Lewy bodies (DLB). Encephalitis could be ruled out because that brain magnetic resonance imaging (MRI) scan didn't show any abnormal signal of inflammation in the brain. In addition, cerebrospinal fluid (CSF) and electroencephalogram (EEG) findings didn't support the possibility of encephalitis as well. In terms of autoimmune encephalopathies, the clinical suspicion was not supported by CSF and serological findings. Moreover, DLB should be differentiated as well. The main manifestations of visual hallucinations,

cognitive dysfunction, and Parkinson-like performance can be found in DLB patients. Patients with DLB may also have sleep problem and autonomic dysfunction. In this case, there were some points that didn't support the diagnosis of DLB. Firstly, there is no report on clustering of DLB in families so far. Secondly, the symptoms of DLB patients are usually fluctuating. Finally, deficit of visuospatial skills is often the prominent feature of cognitive dysfunction in DLB patients. In light of the feature of intractable insomnia and positive family history in this patient, genetic Creutzfeldt–Jakob disease should be considered as the most likely diagnosis. Therefore, the genetic testing was performed to test the preliminary diagnosis.

Additional Tests or Key Results

Genetic testing was performed in the patient during the period of hospitalization, and the results revealed the p.D178N mutation (Fig. 7.14) and 129MM codon (Fig. 7.14) in *PRNP* gene.

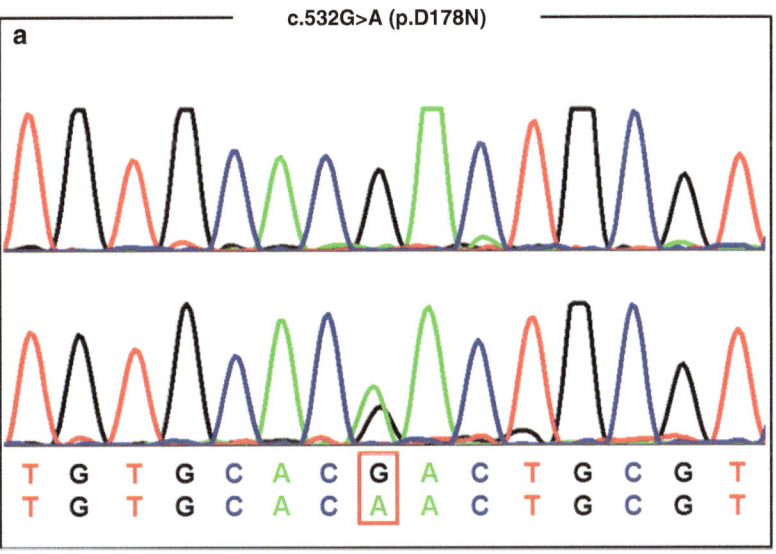

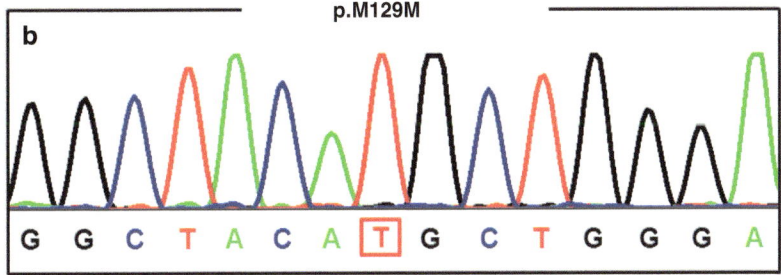

Fig. 7.14 Mutation analysis of the patient. (**a**) Chromatogram of c.532G>A (p.D178N) mutation in *PRNP*. The *upper panel* is normal sequence of the control, whereas the *lower panel* represents heterozygous mutated sequence of the patient. (**b**) Chromatogram of 129 Met homozygous in *PRNP*

Discussion

Fatal familial insomnia (FFI) is a rapidly progressive disease characterized by insomnia, autonomic dysfunction, pyramidal and extrapyramidal signs, and cognitive disturbances. The first description of this disease is credited to Lugaresi in 1986 [46]. FFI is caused by the mutations in the *PRNP* gene and usually inherited in an autosomal dominant pattern. The disease usually occurs between age 20 and 72 years, with the average age of onset of 49.5 years [47]. The duration of the disease is between 5 and 44 months, with a mean duration of 11 months [47]. As one of three genetic prion diseases, FFI is also an extremely rare disease with an incidence estimated at 1/1,000,000. The pathogenesis of FFI is not well understood, though it is believed to be in strong relationship with the amount of conversion from PrP to PrPres protein. But the specific mechanism for the conversion is still unclear.

A wide range of symptoms have been described in FFI patients, and these symptoms vary greatly between FFI patients. Phenotypic variability was believed to relate to the p.M129V polymorphism. Myoclonus, spatial disorientation, and hallucinations were more common symptoms in FFI patients with 129MM genotype, which has been verified in the present case.

But for those patients with 129MV genotype, it is much easier to observe the bulbar disturbances and vegetative dysfunction [48]. Moreover, a shorter average survival time and clinical course were observed in 129MM FFI patients when compared to 129MV FFI patients [49]. A rapid progression of disease with a total of 7 months clinical course was observed in the present case. The possible explanation for the phenotypic variation led by p.M129V polymorphism is the result of different rates of PrPc to PrPSc conversion.

The diagnosis of FFI is mainly based on the careful clinical observation and the significant findings of polysomnography and PET imaging prior to mutation analysis. The sleep problem is the earliest and most prominent manifestation. Polysomnography is critical to the diagnosis of FFI and could provide the evidence of reduced appearance of sleep spindles and *K* complexes. As another useful diagnostic tool, PET could display hypometabolism in the thalamus and cingulate cortex, which is considered the hallmark of FFI. The genetic testing could be the most effective means to help establish the diagnosis of FFI. Currently, there is no effective treatment for FFI, and available drugs are mainly aimed to alleviate symptoms.

7.6   Niemann–Pick Disease (NPD)

A 20-Year-Old Male with Behavioral Abnormalities and Unsteadiness

Clinical Presentations
A 20-year-old male presented with behavioral abnormalities, blurred speech, and unsteadiness. The patient was healthy at birth and grew up with normal developmental milestones. After entering elementary school at 7 years of age, he had no obvious problems with his schoolwork. However, he seemed to show less positive social interaction with classmates and spend more time on his own than with peers. The parents noticed his behavioral problems after he entered high school at 16 years old. He began to talk with himself, yell with meaningless words, and giggle alone. There were no symptoms of headache, double vision, swallowing difficulties, fever, or confusion. There was no history of alcohol excess. He was not on any regular medications. He was brought to the clinic and diagnosed with schizophrenia. After the treatment of antipsychotic drugs, the symptoms were partially alleviated, but the patient still dropped out of the school. The patient had gradually became clumsy in limbs, including writing or grabbing something, with unsteady gait from 17 years of age. The family history was unremarkable and the parents were non-consanguineous (Fig. 7.15).

The examination of cranial nerves revealed a slightly blurred speech and vertical gaze

difficulty. The muscle strength was normal with decreased tone and reflexes. The cerebellar examination revealed bilateral slow alternate movements and moderate dysmetria in the finger-to-nose and heel-to-shin tests. The gait examination revealed a broad-based gait and walking difficulty in a straight line. Only mild cognitive impairment was noted, with the Mini-Mental State Examination (MMSE) score of 26/30 and the Montreal Cognitive Assessment score of 13/30.

Liver and renal function, blood glucose, serum electrolyte, ceruloplasmin, vitamin B12, ammonia, and lactate level were normal. Blood amino acids, acylcarnitine, alpha-fetoprotein, and urinary organic acids were normal. Abdominal ultrasound demonstrated splenomegaly (108*46 mm). Brain MRI showed sporadic focal hyperintensity on T2-weighted and T2-FLAIR images involving frontal and parietal lobes. Electroencephalography was within normal range.

Primary Diagnosis
The history and examinations revealed a cerebellar ataxia with psychiatric symptoms in adolescent or young adult. The differential diagnosis included secondary ataxias (e.g., hypothyroidism, paraneoplastic ataxia, toxics), Wilson's disease (WD), common young–adult-onset autosomal recessive cerebellar ataxia (ARCA) including ataxia with oculomotor apraxia (AOA), Niemann–Pick disease type C (NPC), Refsum disease, GM2 gangliosidosis, Krabbe disease, and rarely autosomal dominant cerebellar ataxia (ADCA) causing by de novo mutations. According to the history and lab tests, we considered ARCA first. Among them, AOA and NPC could affect the movement of eyes, and vertical gaze palsy strongly points toward the diagnosis of NPC.

Additional Tests or Key Results
DNA sequencing found two heterozygous mutations within *NPC1*, c.2366G>A (p.R789H) and c.2972_2973delAG (p.Q991Rfs*15) (Fig. 7.16), with no mutation in *NPC2*. The *NPC1* mutations were confirmed by the analysis of family members.

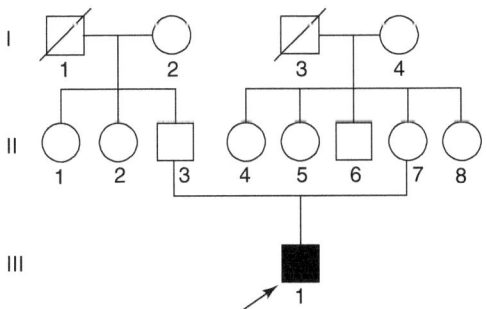

Fig. 7.15 Pedigree of the family. Squares indicate males; circles indicate females; the filled square indicates the affected male; the diagonal lines across symbols indicate the deceased individuals; the arrow indicates the proband

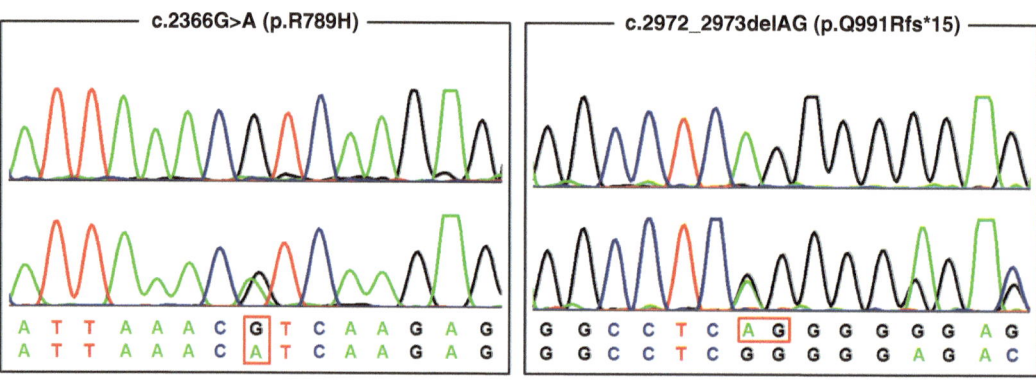

Fig. 7.16 Chromatogram of the c.2366G>A and c.2972_2973delAG mutations within *NPC1*. The *upper panels* are normal sequences, whereas the *lower panels* represent mutated ones

Discussion

Niemann–Pick disease type C (NPC) is an autosomal recessive lysosomal storage disorder caused by mutations in the *NPC1* gene on chromosome 18q11 or *NPC2* gene on chromosome 14q24.3 [49]. The mutations cause impaired cholesterol esterification and lipid trafficking. Unesterified cholesterol and glycolipids accumulate in the lysosome and lead to a vulnerability of the neuronal cells, especially for cerebellar Purkinje cells [51]. The disease can progress slowly and affect older patients up to the fifth decade, but the average age of diagnosis is about 10 years [52].

A variety of phenotypes has been reported with NPC depending on the age of onset of symptoms. The most common neurological manifestations include cerebellar ataxia, vertical supranuclear gaze palsy, dysarthria, cognitive impairment, splenomegaly, and psychiatric disorders, but any of them can be absent [53]. In addition, vertical supranuclear gaze palsy is a relative characteristic clinical sign in NPC patients, as in our patient, but it can also appear in other conditions such as kernicterus and neurodegeneration with brain iron accumulation (NBIA) and spinocerebellar ataxia [54].

Cognitive deficits range from a mild impairment to severe dementia with mutism. Splenomegaly is more common in early-onset patients, with or without hepatomegaly. In older patients, abdominal ultrasound may be required to detect the mild splenomegaly [50]. The splenomegaly is often asymptomatic, as well as in this patient. Cataplexy is a more specific but less frequent symptom in NPC patients. Our patient developed cataplexy in the follow-up.

Juvenile patients with early cognitive decline and/or psychosis can be very challenging to diagnose, because the phenotypes are nonspecific which can be erroneously attributed to developmental delay or to autism/schizophrenia as seen in this patient, particularly when treatment of antipsychotics has been started, and side effects may mask disease-related movement disorders [55].

The *NPC1/NPC2* gene mutation testing is confirmatory. About 95% of patients have mutations in the *NPC1* gene. Skin, liver, and bone marrow biopsy as well as filipin staining may be supportive but not specific. Oxysterols (cholesterol oxidation products) may be excellent markers for screening of NPC [50].

NPC is not associated with pathognomonic features on neuroimaging assessment [50]. The common changes on brain magnetic resonance imaging (MRI) include mild or considerable generalized cortical atrophy and multiple non-enhancing hyperintense areas in the periventricular white matter on T2-weighted images in a pattern that resembles multiple sclerosis (MS), which is consistent with observation in this patient [53, 56].

The prognosis of NPC is poor, and individualized symptomatic treatments are recommended. Miglustat, an inhibitor of glucosylceramide synthase, is the only disease-specific drug approved for the treatment of progressive neurological manifestations in NPC patients [50].

In summary, the diagnosis of NPC is challenging due to the heterogeneous nature of the clinical phenotypes. The combinations of the symptoms/signs (ataxia, psychotic symptoms, vertical gaze palsy, splenomegaly, cataplexy) may suggest the diagnosis, and genetic testing is confirmatory.

References

1. Bauer P, Laccone F, Rolfs A, Wüllner U, Bösch S, Peters H, Liebscher S, Scheible M, Epplen J, Weber B. Trinucleotide repeat expansion in SCA17/TBP in white patients with Huntington's disease-like phenotype. J Med Genet. 2004;41(3):230–2.

2. Rolfs A, Koeppen AH, Bauer I, Bauer P, Buhlmann S, Topka H, Schöls L, Riess O. Clinical features and neuropathology of autosomal dominant spinocerebellar ataxia (SCA17). Ann Neurol. 2003;54(3):367–75.

3. Kanazawa I. Dentatorubral-pallidoluysian atrophy or Naito-Oyanagi disease. Neurogenetics. 1998; 2(1):1–17.

4. Paleacu D, Schechtman E, Inzelberg R. Association between family history of dementia and hallucinations in Parkinson disease. Neurology. 2005;64(10): 1712–5.

5. Bates GP, Dorsey R, Gusella JF, Hayden MR, Kay C, Leavitt BR, Nance M, Ross CA, Scahill RI, Wetzel R. Huntington disease. Nat Rev Dis Primers. 2015;1:15005.

6. Schoenfeld M, Myers RH, Cupples LA, Berkman B, Sax DS, Clark E. Increased rate of suicide among patients with Huntington's disease. J Neurol Neurosurg Psychiatry. 1984;47(12):1283–7.

7. Huntington G. On chorea. Med Surg Report Weekly J (Philadelphia: S.W. Butler). 1872;26(15):317–21.

8. Group HsDCR. A novel gene containing a trinucleotide repeat that is expanded and unstable on Huntington's disease chromosomes. Cell. 1993;72:971–83.

9. Bean L, Bayrak-Toydemir P, Committee ALQA. American College of Medical Genetics and Genomics Standards and Guidelines for Clinical Genetics Laboratories, 2014 edition: technical standards and guidelines for Huntington disease. Genet Med. 2014;16(12):e2.

10. Lee J-M, Ramos E, Lee J-H, Gillis T, Mysore J, Hayden M, Warby S, Morrison P, Nance M, Ross C. CAG repeat expansion in Huntington disease determines age at onset in a fully dominant fashion. Neurology. 2012;78(10):690–5.

11. Wexler NS. Venezuelan kindreds reveal that genetic and environmental factors modulate Huntington's disease age of onset. Proc Natl Acad Sci U S A. 2004;101(10):3498–503.

12. Milunsky J, Maher T, Loose B, Darras B, Ito M. XL PCR for the detection of large trinucleotide expansions in juvenile Huntington's disease. Clin Genet. 2003;64(1):70–3.

13. Rosenblatt A. Neuropsychiatry of Huntington's disease. Dialogues Clin Neurosci. 2007;9(2):191–7.

14. Duff K, Paulsen JS, Beglinger LJ, Langbehn DR, Stout JC. Group P-HIotHS. Psychiatric symptoms in Huntington's disease before diagnosis: the predict-HD study. Biol Psychiatry. 2007;62(12):1341–6.

15. Gatto EM, Parisi V, Etcheverry JL, Sanguinetti A, Cordi L, Binelli A, Persi G, Squitieri F. Juvenile Huntington disease in Argentina. Arq Neuropsiquiatr. 2016;74(1):50–4.

16. Henley SM, Wild EJ, Hobbs NZ, Warren JD, Frost C, Scahill RI, Ridgway GR, MacManus DG, Barker RA, Fox NC. Defective emotion recognition in early HD is neuropsychologically and anatomically generic. Neuropsychologia. 2008;46(8):2152–60.

17. Shannon KM, Fraint A. Therapeutic advances in Huntington's disease. Mov Disord. 2015;30(11): 1539–46.

18. Nance M, Paulsen JS, Rosenblatt A, Wheelock V. A Physician's guide to the management of Huntington's disease. New York: Huntington's Disease Society of America; 2015.

19. Chabriat H, Vahedi K, Iba-Zizen MT, Joutel A, Nibbio A, Nagy TG, Krebs MO, Julien J, Dubois B, Ducrocq X, et al. Clinical spectrum of CADASIL: a study of 7 families. Cerebral autosomal dominant arteriopathy with subcortical infarcts and leukoencephalopathy. Lancet. 1995;346(8980):934–9.

20. Joutel A, Corpechot C, Ducros A, Vahedi K, Chabriat H, Mouton P, Alamowitch S, Domenga V, Cecillion M, Marechal E, Maciazek J, Vayssiere C, Cruaud C, Cabanis EA, Ruchoux MM, Weissenbach J, Bach JF, Bousser MG, Tournier-Lasserve E. Notch3 mutations in CADASIL, a hereditary adult-onset condition causing stroke and dementia. Nature. 1996;383(6602):707–10.

21. Federico A, Bianchi S, Dotti MT. The spectrum of mutations for CADASIL diagnosis. Neurol Sci. 2005;26(2):117–24.

22. Wang Z, Yuan Y, Zhang W, Lv H, Hong D, Chen B, Liu Y, Luan X, Xie S, Wu S. NOTCH3 mutations and clinical features in 33 mainland Chinese families with CADASIL. J Neurol Neurosurg Psychiatry. 2011;82(5):534–9.

23. Liu X, Zuo Y, Sun W, Zhang W, Lv H, Huang Y, Xiao J, Yuan Y, Wang Z. The genetic spectrum and the evaluation of CADASIL screening scale in Chinese patients with NOTCH3 mutations. J Neurol Sci. 2015;354(1–2):63–9.

24. Liao YC, Hsiao CT, Fuh JL, Chern CM, Lee WJ, Guo YC, Wang SJ, Lee IH, Liu YT, Wang YF, Chang FC, Chang MH, Soong BW, Lee YC. Characterization of CADASIL among the Han Chinese in Taiwan: Distinct Genotypic and Phenotypic Profiles. PLoS One. 2015;10(8):e0136501.

25. Chabriat H, Joutel A, Dichgans M, Tournier-Lasserve E, Bousser MG. Cadasil. Lancet Neurol. 2009;8(7):643–53.

26. Markus HS, Martin RJ, Simpson MA, Dong YB, Ali N, Crosby AH, Powell JF. Diagnostic strategies in CADASIL. Neurology. 2002;59(8):1134–8.

27. Tikka S, Mykkanen K, Ruchoux MM, Bergholm R, Junna M, Poyhonen M, Yki-Jarvinen H, Joutel A, Viitanen M, Baumann M, Kalimo H. Congruence between NOTCH3 mutations and GOM in 131 CADASIL patients. Brain. 2009;132(Pt 4):933–9.

28. Yanagawa S, Ito N, Arima K, et al. Cerebral autosomal recessive arteriopathy with subcortical infarcts andleukoencephalopathy. Neurology. 2002;58(5):817–20.

29. Nozaki H, Nishizawa M, Onodera O. Features of cerebral autosomal recessive ArteriopathyWith subcortical infarcts and leukoencephalopathy. Stroke. 2014;45(11):3447–53.

30. Wang XL, Li CF, Guo HW, et al. A novel mutation in the HTRA1 gene identified in Chinese CARASIL pedigree. CNS Neurosci Ther. 2012;18(10):867–9.

31. Cai B, Zeng JB, Lin Y, et al. A frameshift mutation in HTRA1 expands CARASIL syndrome and peripheral small arterial disease to the Chinese population. Neurol Sci. 2015;36(8):1387–91.

32. Mendioroz M, Fernandez-Cadenas I, Del RA, et al. A missense HTRA1 mutation expands CARASIL syndrome to the Caucasian population. Neurology. 2010;75(22):2033–5.

33. Bianchi S, Di PC, Gallus GN, et al. Two novel HTRA1 mutations in a European CARASIL patient. Neurology. 2014;82(10):898–900.

34. Hara K, Shiga A, Fukutake T, et al. Association of HTRA1 mutations and familial ischemic cerebral small-vesseldisease. N Engl J Med. 2009;360(17):1729–39.

35. Fukutake T. Cerebral autosomal recessive arteriopathy with subcortical infarcts andleukoencephalopathy (CARASIL): from discovery to gene identification. J Stroke Cerebrovasc Dis. 2011;20(2):85–93.

36. Oide T, Nakayama H, Yanagawa S, et al. Extensive loss of arterial medial smooth muscle cells and mural extracellularmatrix in cerebral autosomal recessive arteriopathy with subcortical infarcts andleukoencephalopathy (CARASIL). Neuropathology. 2008;28(2):132–42.

37. Cai B, Lin Y, Xue XH, et al. TAT-mediated delivery of neuroglobin protects against focal cerebral ischemia in mice. Exp Neurol. 2011;227(1):224–31.

38. Bezman L, Moser AB, Raymond GV, Rinaldo P, Watkins PA, Smith KD, Kass NE, Moser HW. Adrenoleukodystrophy: incidence, new mutation rate, and results of extended family screening. Ann Neurol. 2001;49(4):512–7.

39. Kemp S, Valianpour F, Denis S, Ofman R, Sanders RJ, Mooyer P, Barth PG, Wanders RJ. Elongation of very long-chain fatty acids is enhanced in X-linked adrenoleukodystrophy. Mol Genet Metab. 2005;84(2):144–51.

40. Mosser J, Douar AM, Sarde CO, Kioschis P, Feil R, Moser H, Poustka AM, Mandel JL, Aubourg P. Putative X-linked adrenoleukodystrophy gene shares unexpected homology with ABC transporters. Nature. 1993;361(6414):726–30.

41. Kok F, Neumann S, Sarde CO, Zheng S, Wu KH, Wei HM, Bergin J, Watkins PA, Gould S, Sack G, et al. Mutational analysis of patients with X-linked adrenoleukodystrophy. Hum Mutat. 1995;6(2):104–15.

42. Kemp S, Pujol A, Waterham HR, van Geel BM, Boehm CD, Raymond GV, Cutting GR, Wanders RJ, Moser HW. ABCD1 mutations and the X-linked adrenoleukodystrophy mutation database: role in diagnosis and clinical correlations. Hum Mutat. 2001;18(6):499–515.

43. Moser HW, Loes DJ, Melhem ER, Raymond GV, Bezman L, Cox CS, Lu SE. X-linked adrenoleukodystrophy: overview and prognosis as a function of age and brain magnetic resonance imaging abnormality. A study involving 372 patients. Neuropediatrics. 2000;31(5):227–39.

44. Steinberg SJ, Moser AB, Raymond GV. X-linked adrenoleukodystrophy. In: Pagon RA, Adam MP, Ardinger HH, Wallace SE, Amemiya A, Bean LJH, Bird TD, Ledbetter N, Mefford HC, Smith RJH, Stephens K, eds. GeneReviews® [Internet]. Seattle (WA): University of Washington, Seattle; 1993–2017. 1999 Mar 26 [updated 2015 Apr 9].

45. Engelen M, Kemp S, de Visser M, van Geel BM, Wanders RJ, Aubourg P, Poll-The BT. X-linked adrenoleukodystrophy (X-ALD): clinical presentation and guidelines for diagnosis, follow-up and management. Orphanet J Rare Dis. 2012;7:51.

46. Lugaresi E, Medori R, Montagna P, et al. Fatal familial insomnia and dysautonomia with selective degeneration of thalamic nuclei. N Engl J Med. 1986;315(16):997–1003.

47. Harder A, Gregor A, Wirth T, et al. Early age of onset in fatal familial insomnia. Two novel cases and review of the literature. J Neurol. 2004;251(6):715–24.

48. Krasnianski A, Bartl M, Sanchez Juan PJ, et al. Fatal familial insomnia: clinical features and early identification. Ann Neurol. 2008;63(5):658–61.

49. Montagna P, Cortelli P, Avoni P, et al. Clinical features of fatal familial insomnia: phenotypic variability in relation to a polymorphism at codon 129 of the prion protein gene. Brain Pathol. 1998;8:515–20.

50. Patterson MC, Hendriksz CJ, Walterfang M, Sedel F, Vanier MT, Wijburg F, Group N-CGW. Recommendations for the diagnosis and management of Niemann-

Pick disease type C: an update. Mol Genet Metab. 2012;106(3):330–44.

51. Sturley SL, Patterson MC, Balch W, Liscum L. The pathophysiology and mechanisms of NP-C disease. Biochim Biophys Acta. 2004;1685(1–3):83–7.

52. Sevin M, Lesca G, Baumann N, Millat G, Lyon-Caen O, Vanier MT, Sedel F. The adult form of Niemann-Pick disease type C. Brain. 2007;130(Pt 1):120–33.

53. Lazzaro VD, Marano M, Florio L, De Santis S. Niemann-Pick type C: focus on the adolescent/adult onset form. Int J Neurosci. 2016;126(11):963–71.

54. Salsano E, Umeh C, Rufa A, Pareyson D, Zee DS. Vertical supranuclear gaze palsy in Niemann-Pick type C disease. Neurol Sci. 2012;33(6): 1225–32.

55. Bauer P, Balding DJ, Klunemann HH, Linden DE, Ory DS, Pineda M, Priller J, Sedel F, Muller A, Chadha-Boreham H, Welford RW, Strasser DS, Patterson MC. Genetic screening for Niemann-Pick disease type C in adults with neurological and psychiatric symptoms: findings from the ZOOM study. Hum Mol Genet. 2013;22(21):4349–56.

56. Grau AJ, Brandt T, Weisbrod M, Niethammer R, Forsting M, Cantz M, Vanier MT, Harzer K. Adult Niemann-Pick disease type C mimicking features of multiple sclerosis. J Neurol Neurosurg Psychiatry. 1997;63(4):552.